Pocketbook of Taping Techniques

Commissioning Editor: Rita Demetriou-Swanwick
Development Editors: Veronika Watkins, Louisa Welch
Project Manager: Elouise Ball
Designer/Design Direction: Charles Gray
Illustration Manager: Gillian Richards

Pocketbook of Taping Techniques

Edited by

Rose Macdonald BA FCSP
Consultant in Sports Physiotherapy, Former Director, Sports Injury Centre,
Crystal Palace National Sports Centre, London, UK

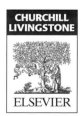

CHURCHILL
LIVINGSTONE

ELSEVIER

Edinburgh   London   New York   Oxford   Philadelphia   St Louis   Sydney   Toronto   2010

CHURCHILL
LIVINGSTONE
ELSEVIER

First published 2010, © Elsevier Limited. All rights reserved.

No part of this publication may be reproduced or transmitted in any form or by any means, electronic or mechanical, including photocopying, recording, or any information storage and retrieval system, without permission in writing from the publisher. Permissions may be sought directly from Elsevier's Rights Department: phone: (+1) 215 239 3804 (US) or (+44) 1865 843830 (UK); fax: (+44) 1865 853333; e-mail: healthpermissions@elsevier.com. You may also complete your request online via the Elsevier website at http://www.elsevier.com/permissions.

ISBN 978-0-7020-3027-7

British Library Cataloguing in Publication Data
A catalogue record for this book is available from the British Library

Library of Congress Cataloging in Publication Data
A catalog record for this book is available from the Library of Congress

Notice
Knowledge and best practice in this field are constantly changing. As new research and experience broaden our knowledge, changes in practice, treatment and drug therapy may become necessary or appropriate. Readers are advised to check the most current information provided (i) on procedures featured or (ii) by the manufacturer of each product to be administered, to verify the recommended dose or formula, the method and duration of administration, and contraindications. It is the responsibility of the practitioner, relying on their own experience and knowledge of the patient, to make diagnoses, to determine dosages and the best treatment for each individual patient, and to take all appropriate safety precautions. To the fullest extent of the law, neither the Publisher nor the Editor assumes any liability for any injury and/or damage to persons or property arising out of or related to any use of the material contained in this book.

The Publisher

ELSEVIER your source for books,
journals and multimedia
in the health sciences

www.elsevierhealth.com

Working together to grow
libraries in developing countries

www.elsevier.com | www.bookaid.org | www.sabre.org

 ELSEVIER BOOK AID International Sabre Foundation

The
Publisher's
policy is to use
**paper manufactured
from sustainable forests**

Printed in China

Contents

Contents

Contents

This book is dedicated to the memory of Ian,
my ever-loving soulmate.

Contributors

Chuck Armstrong
MScPT MEd

Armstrong's Physiotherapy Clinic, Saskatoon, Canada

Michael J Callaghan
Phd Mphil MCSP SRP

Centre for Rehabilitation Science, Manchester Royal Infirmary, Manchester, UK

Wayne A Hing
Msc(Hons) ADP(OMt) DipMT DipPhys

School of Physiotherapy, Auckland University of Technology, Auckland, New Zealand

Andrew Hughes
BAppSc(Phty) MAPA FASMF

Sports Focus Physiotherapy, Liverpool, New South Wales, Australia

David Kneeshaw
BAppSc(Phty) MAPA

Balmain Physiotherapy and Sports, Injury Centre, Balmain, New South Wales, Australia

Gary Lapenskie
BSc(PE) BSC(PT) MA(PE)

Faculty of Kinesiology, University of Western Ontario, London, Ontario, Canada

Ulrik McCarthy Persson
PhD MSc MMACP MISCP

College Lecturer and Course Director (Sports Physiotherapy), UCD School of Physiotherapy and Performance Science, Dublin, Ireland

Jenny McConnell
BAppSci(Phty) GradDipManTher MBiomedEng

McConnell and Clements Physiotherapy, Mosman, New South Wales, Australia

Rose Macdonald
BA FCSP

Consultant in Sports Physiotherapy, London, UK

Helen Millson
M(Phil) Sports Physiotherapy UCT MCSP

IPRS Ltd., Little Blakenham, Suffolk, UK

Dylan Morrissey
PhD MSc BSc(Hons) MMACP MCSP

Consultant Physiotherapist, Tower Hamlets Primary Care Trust, London, UK
Senior Clinical Lecturer in Sports and Exercise Medicine, Barts and The London
School of Medicine and Dentistry, Queen Mary, University of London, London, UK

Jeff O' Neill
MS ATC

Miami, Florida, USA

Dale Reese
BSc

Medicinskt Centrum Norrköping, Norrköping, Sweden

Duncan A Reid
BSc DipPhys DipMT PGD(Manips) MNZCP

School of Physiotherapy, Auckland University of Technology, Auckland,
New Zealand

Olivier Rouillon
MD

Ormesson-sur-marne, France

Kenneth E Wright
DA ATC MHSc PGD(ManipPhys) DipMT DipPhys BSc

Department of Health Sciences, University of Alabama, Tuscaloosa, Alabama, USA

Preface

Taping is now recognized as a skill which is essential for all those involved in the treatment and rehabilitation of injuries. It is widely used not only for sports injuries, but also for many other conditions such as muscle imbalance, unstable joints and impaired neural control. During treatment and rehabilitation, taping aids the healing process by supporting and protecting the injured structures from further injury or stress, thus reducing the need for prolonged treatment and time off work.

New techniques are constantly being developed for injury *prevention* which may also be used in general practice and in the hospital environment for the non-sporting population. Once the basic techniques are mastered, then it is up to the practitioners to modify, change and develop new techniques themselves, always adhering to taping principles.

To aid in the development of new techniques, this pocketbook has many new ideas which may be used as indicated or modified to suit the situation. Many of the 'old favourites' are included, as basic techniques are fundamental to the practice of good taping. Chapters on techniques to alter muscle activity and proprioception, with scientific evidence, are also included for those not familiar with this type of taping.

Sports medicine leans towards early mobilization through functional therapy, and total immobilization in plaster casts is becoming less common. Removable cast bracing is used instead, to enable therapy to continue throughout the recovery phase. Taping a limb or body part is like applying a 'flexible cast' which aids in the prevention of further injury and rests the affected part. Flexible tape casts limit the range of motion and may be used in many sports where rigid supports are not allowed.

On some occasions a bandage is more appropriate than tape. Therefore, at the end of this pocketbook, as an aide memoire, there are two short sections on spica (figure-of-eight) bandaging and the construction of arm slings using a triangular bandage.

New contributors from South Africa, Ireland and the UK share their expertise, bringing an abundant array of new evidence-based techniques and updated literature to the pocketbook.

Rose Macdonald 2009

Acknowledgements

First, I wish to thank all the contributors for sharing their proven techniques with us, and for their cooperation and patience.

I should also like to thank Churchill Livingstone for inviting me to compile and edit this new *Pocketbook of Taping Techniques*. I am grateful to their production team for designing the layout of the book in such a way that the text and diagrams are easy to follow and understand at a glance.

I should especially like to thank the Elsevier team, Veronika Watkins, Rita Demetriou-Swanwick and Louisa Welch for their help in steering me through the process of putting this new pocketbook together.

Thank you to St John Ambulance for kindly allowing their diagrams to be used again as an 'aide memoire'.

part 1

PART CONTENTS

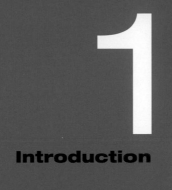

1 chapter

Introduction

R. Macdonald

CHAPTER CONTENTS

The application of tape to injured soft tissues and joints provides support and protection for these structures and minimizes pain and swelling in the acute stage. Tape should reinforce the normal supportive structures in their relaxed position and protect the injured tissues from further damage. Many different techniques are used for injury prevention, treatment, rehabilitation, proprioception and sport.

Various techniques are illustrated in this manual, together with different philosophies expressed by the contributors – many of whom are eminent physical therapists in their respective countries.

ROLE OF TAPING

Initially, tape is applied to protect the injured structure during the treatment and rehabilitation programme:

- to hold dressings and pads in place
- to compress recent injury, thus reducing bleeding and swelling
- to protect from further injury by supporting ligaments, tendons and muscles
- to limit unwanted joint movement
- to allow optimal healing without stressing the injured structures
- to protect and support the injured structure in a functional position during the exercise, strengthening and proprioceptive programme.

It must be clearly understood that taping is not a substitute for treatment and rehabilitation, but is an adjunct to the total injury-care programme.

TYPES OF TAPE

Good-quality tape should adhere readily and maintain adhesion despite perspiration and activity.

Stretch adhesive tape (elastic adhesive bandage, EAB)

Conforms to the contours of the body, allowing for normal tissue expansion, and is used for the following:

- to compress and support soft tissue
- to provide anchors around muscle, thus allowing for expansion
- to hold protective pads in place.

Stretch tape will not give mechanical support to ligaments, but may be used in conjunction with rigid tape to give added support. Stretch tape is not normally tearable and must be cut with scissors, but there are now available very light-weight stretch tapes which may be torn by hand. Stretch tape is available in a variety of widths, from 1.25 to 10 cm, and sometimes even wider. Stretch tape may have:

- one-way stretch, in length *or* width
- two-way stretch, in length *and* width.

Stretch tape tends to roll back on itself at the cut ends, therefore it is wise to allow the last couple of centimetres to recoil before sticking it down.

Non-stretch adhesive tape

Has a non-yielding cloth backing and is used for the following:

- to support inert structures, e.g. ligaments, joint capsule
- to limit joint movement
- to act prophylactically
- to secure the ends of stretch tape
- to reinforce stretch tape
- to enhance proprioception.

Non-stretch tape should be torn by hand to maintain tension during application. It is important to be able to tear the tape from various positions – practice will help to attain a high level of efficiency.

Note: Leukotape P is an extra-strong non-stretch adhesive tape.

Tearing technique

Tear the tape close to the roll, keeping it taut. Hold the tape with the thumb and index fingers close together. Rip the tape quickly in scissors fashion. Practise tearing a strip of tape into very small pieces in both directions, lengthwise and crossways.

Hypoallergenic tapes

Hypafix/Fixomull offer an alternative to conventional zinc oxide adhesive tape, to which some athletes are allergic.

Waterproof tape

Also available in many widths.

Cohesive bandages

Are a useful product and may be used instead of stretch tape. The product sticks to itself and not to the skin, is waterproof and is reusable.

These are most useful when applying spica bandages or as a cover-up for any tape procedure.

TAPING PRINCIPLES

The application of tape is easy, but if it is not carried out correctly it will be of little value and may even be detrimental. Therefore knowledge of the basic principles and practical aspects is essential if the full value of the technique is to be attained.

A thorough assessment is necessary before taping any structure. The following questions should be answered:

• Has the injury been thoroughly assessed?
• How did the injury occur?
• What structures were damaged?
• What tissues need protection and support?
• What movements must be restricted?
• Is the injury acute or chronic?
• Is immobilization necessary at this stage?
• Are you familiar with the anatomy and biomechanics of the parts involved?
• Can you visualize the purpose for which the tape is to be applied?
• Are you familiar with the technique?
• Do you have suitable materials at hand?

Notes

If you are considering taping a player on the field, ensure that the use of tape does not contravene the rules of the sport, thus making the player ineligible to participate. *Know the sport.* Is there time allowed for taping on the field? Or do you have to remove the player from the field of play in order to apply tape? You must also consider the event in which the athlete is participating.

TAPING GUIDELINES

Prepare the area to be taped:
• Wash, dry and shave the skin in a downward direction.
• Remove oils for better adhesion.
• Cover broken lesions before taping; an electric shaver avoids cutting the skin.
• Check if the athlete is allergic to tape or spray.
• Apply lubricated protective padding to friction and pressure areas.

- Apply adhesive spray for skin protection and better tape adhesion.
- Apply underwrap for sensitive skin.

Tips

If the area is frequently taped, move the anchor point on successive tapings to prevent skin irritation.

Tape application

- Have all the required materials at hand.
- Have the athlete and yourself in a comfortable position, e.g. couch at an optimal working height, to avoid fatigue.
- Apply tape to skin which is at room temperature.
- Have the full attention of the athlete.
- Place the joint in a functional position, with minimum stress on the injured structure.
- Ensure that the ligaments are in the shortened position.
- Use the correct type, width and amount of tape for the procedure.
- Apply strips of tape in a sequential order.
- Overlap successive strips by half to prevent slippage and gapping.
- Apply each strip with a particular purpose in mind.
- Apply tape smoothly and firmly.
- Flow with the shape of the limb.
- Explain the function of the tape to the athlete, and how it should feel.
- On completion, check that the tape is functional and comfortable.

The tape should conform with even pressure and must be effective and comfortable. Tape applied directly to the skin gives maximum support.

Tips

For acutely angled areas, rip the tape longitudinally into strips. Small strips are easier to conform by lapping them over each other.

Avoid

- excessive traction on skin – this may lead to skin breakdown
- gaps and wrinkles – these may cause blisters
- continuous circumferential taping – single strips produce a more uniform pressure

- excessive layers of tape – this may impair circulation and neural transmission
- too tight an application over bony areas – this may cause bone ache.

Tape removal

Never rip tape off, especially from the plantar aspect of the foot. Use a tape cutter or bandage scissors for safe, fast removal. Lubricate the tip with petroleum jelly and slide it parallel to the skin in the natural soft-tissue channels.

Remove the tape carefully by peeling it back on itself, and pushing the skin away from the tape. Pull the tape carefully along the axis of the limb.

Check the skin for damage and apply lotion to restore skin moisture. Tape should not be left on for more than 24 h, unless using hypoallergenic tape which may be left on longer. Leaving tape on for too long a period may lead to skin breakdown.

Return to activity

On return to activity the injured area is still at risk. Reinjury can be prevented by taping the weakened area, with the aim of restricting joint and muscle movement to within safe limits. This allows performance with confidence.

Lax and hypermobile joints may also be supported with adhesive tape in order to reduce the risk of injury during sport.

STORAGE

Tape with zinc oxide adhesive mass is susceptible to temperature change and should be stored in a cool place. Tape should be left in its original packing until required. Partially used rolls should be kept in an airtight container (e.g. cooler box or plastic box) and not left on shelves. At temperatures over 20°C the adhesive mass becomes sticky, making the tension stronger and thus more difficult to unwind. Non-stretch tape is also more difficult to tear when warm. Hypoallergenic tapes are not susceptible to temperature change.

TAPING TERMS

Anchors: the first strips of tape applied above and below the injury site, and to which subsequent strips are attached. Anchors minimize traction on the skin (skin drag) and are applied without tension.
Support strips and stirrups restrict unwanted sideways movement.
Gibney/horizontal strips add stability to the joint.

Reinforcing strips restrict movement and add tensile strength to strategic areas when applied over stretch tape.

Check reins restrict range of motion.

Lock strips secure the cut end of stretch tape (which tends to roll back on itself), secure check reins in place, and neatly finish the technique when applied over anchors (fill strips).

Heel locks give additional support to the subtalar and ankle joints.

OTHER TAPING PRODUCTS

Underwrap/prowrap/Mefix/Hypafix/Fixomull: used to protect sensitive skin from zinc oxide adhesive mass.

Gauze squares: foam squares, or heel-and-lace pads, are used to protect areas which are susceptible to stress and friction.

Padding: felt, foam, rubber or other materials for protecting sensitive areas.

Adhesive spray: applied to make skin tacky and thus help underwrap, protective pads or tape adhere more readily.

Friars' Balsam: applied to protect the skin.

Dehesive spray: breaks down the adhesive mass and allows tape to be removed easily.

Tape remover: available as spray, solution or wipes to clean adhesive residue from the skin.

Petroleum jelly: applied to lubricate areas of stress and reduce friction and irritation to the soft tissues.

Talcum powder: used to remove adhesive residue where necessary; it also prevents stretch tape from rolling at the edges.

Cohesive bandage: adheres to itself but not to the skin and can be used for light compression or applied over tape to prevent unravelling in water.

Tubular bandage: may be applied over completed tape job to help set the tape and hold it in place.

Elastic bandage/tensor: used for compression and for traditional spicas.

Cloth wrap: used for ankle wraps, triangular bandages, collar and cuff support.

Tape cutter: allows quick and safe removal of tape.

Bandage scissors: flat-ended scissors for safe removal of tape.

Other useful products

A variety of athletic braces and supports for body parts, neoprene/elastic/other sleeves, rubber tubing, extra long tensor/cohesive bandages for spicas, hot/cold packs, second-skin/blister kit.

2

chapter
◀◀

Taping literature update

M.J. Callaghan

CHAPTER CONTENTS

INTRODUCTION

Taping continues to be an essential part of a physiotherapist's armamentarium in the various stages of rehabilitation after injury and return to competition. Indeed, many athletes consider taping such an essential part of their sporting preparation that it becomes a ritualistic process, occasionally verging on the superstitious! This should not distract us from continuing to investigate the scientific rationale behind its application from the growing wealth of literature. This chapter deals with the literature concerning both ankle taping and patellar taping.

ANKLE TAPING

The literature on ankle taping is considerable, mainly because ankles are easily studied by X-ray, electromyography, goniometry and kinetic and kinematic analysis. The rationale for ankle taping mainly involves treatment after acute injury, mechanical instability and functional instability and injury prevention.

Acute injury

After an acute ligament sprain of the ankle, compressive strapping is often recommended to control oedema (McCluskey et al 1976). Very few studies have been published to evaluate the efficacy of taping to achieve limb or joint compression, with Viljakka (1986) and Rucinski et al (1991) arriving at conflicting conclusions as to the effect of bandaging on acute ankle oedema. Two Cochrane reviews have helped in our understanding of the best approach for treating acute ankle sprains. First, Kerkhoffs et al (2002a) analysed results from 21 trials of acceptable quality. They provided clear overall evidence that it is better, in terms of return to work and sport, pain, swelling, instability, range of motion and recurrence of sprain, for patients to be treated with various ankle braces or supports rather than total immobilization. A second Cochrane review (Kerkhoffs et al 2002b) then tried to give some insight into the best type of brace to use after an acute ankle sprain. However, in nine trials of moderate quality they found that a lace-up brace was superior to a semi-rigid support, tubigrip-type stocking and taping in terms of reduced swelling, but that a semi-rigid brace was superior for quicker return to work and reported ankle instability. This less compelling evidence means that we are unsure of the best type of bracing or support.

Mechanical instability

Preventing extremes of range of movement and reducing the abnormal movement of the ankle are the most obvious roles of ankle taping. In normal subjects, tape has been demonstrated to reduce extremes of ankle range of movement after 15 minutes of running round a figure-of-eight course (Laughman et al 1980). In patients with proven mechanical ankle instability, a zinc oxide Gibney basketweave technique significantly decreased the amount of non-weight-bearing talar tilt (Larsen 1984, Vaes et al 1985). It was noted that those patients with the greatest instability received the greatest benefit from the tape.

Although taping does seem to improve mechanical instability, it is important to note that the restricting effect is lost after varying periods of exercise. For example, 40% of the effect of taping was lost after 10 minutes of vigorous general circuit exercises (Rarick et al 1962). Approximately 50% was lost after 15 minutes of standard vigorous exercises (Frankeny et al 1993), there was a 20% decrease after 20 minutes of stop/start running (Larsen 1984), 37% loosening in total passive range of motion after 20 minutes of volleyball training (Greene & Hillman 1990), 10–20% restriction loss in all movements except dorsiflexion after 60 minutes of squash (Myburgh et al 1984) and a 14% loss of inversion restriction after 30 minutes of exercise (Alt et al 1999). It has also been found that the greater the subject's weight, height and body mass index, the less effective the tape is in controlling supination and ankle plantarflexion after 30 minutes of exercise (Meana et al 2007).

It is this inability to maintain mechanical stability during exercise that raises fundamental questions about the theories behind ankle taping and bracing.

Functional instability

Freeman et al (1965) seem to be among the first to describe functional instability as 'a term ... to designate the disability to which the patients refer when they say that their foot tends to "give way"'. Although once of secondary importance to mechanical problems, there is now more interest in the concept of functional instability of the ankle and the role of taping and bracing to alleviate it. As a result, for many years authors have investigated the role of taping and bracing on the proprioception enhancement of the chronically injured ankle (Glick et al 1976, Hamill et al 1986, Jerosch et al 1995, Karlsson & Andreasson 1992, Lentell et al 1995, Robbins et al 1995).

Proprioceptive control of the ankle (and thus the effect of taping and bracing) has been measured by a variety of tests, such as peroneal reflex activity (Ashton-Miller et al 1996, Feuerbach et al 1994, Karlsson & Andreasson 1992, Konradsen & Hojsgaard 1993, Konradsen et al 1993, Lohrer et al 1999), joint angle reproduction (Jerosch et al 1995, Lentell et al 1995, Refshauge et al 2000, Spanos et al 2008) and movement threshold (Konradsen et al 2000).

Injury prevention

Epidemiological studies have established the ability of tape and braces to prevent recurrent ankle injury. The most commonly cited study on injury prevention is that of Garrick & Requa (1973), which studied the effect of taping on 2563 basketball players with previous ankle sprains over two successive seasons. They concluded that a zinc oxide stirrup with horseshoe and figure-of-eight technique, in combination with a high-top shoe, had a protective influence (6.5 injuries per 1000 games) for preventing ankle sprains.

Ankle braces may also lead to a reduction in the incidence and severity of acute ankle sprains in competition (Bahr 2001), such as basketball (Sitler et al 1994), men's football (soccer) (Surve et al 1994, Tropp et al 1985) and women's football (Sharpe et al 1997). Although the studies reviewed provide important information regarding efficacy of tape or a brace, criticisms have been made regarding study design, external validity, confounding variables and sample size (Sitler et al 1994). These should also be considered before selecting the appropriate technique or device.

A Cochrane review (Handoll et al 2001) summarized the relative risk of ankle sprains after application of braces and calculated that ankle bracing brought about a 50% reduction in the number of ankle sprains (relative risk (RR) = 0.53). The reduction was greatest for patients with previous ankle sprains.

Prewrap

Two studies have looked at the effects of prewrap on taping that may ease the reservations among clinicians of the effects of prewrap or underwrap on taping. Manfroy et al (1997) assessed 20 healthy subjects performing 40 minutes of exercise and found no statistically significant differences in experimental limitation of inversion moments between ankle taping with and without prewrap. Ricard et al (2000) measured the amount and rate of dynamic ankle inversion using a trapdoor inversion platform apparatus and concluded that applying tape over prewrap was as effective as applying it directly to skin.

Taping technique

The lack of comparative studies between different taping techniques helps to explain why the choice of tape by athletes and physiotherapists is often governed by personal preference, the experience of the person applying the tape and a general feel as to the correct technique.

Of those few studies, Rarick et al (1962) favoured a basketweave with stirrup and heel-lock technique. Frankeny et al (1993) concluded that the Hinton–Boswell method (in which the ankle is taped in a relaxed plantarflexed position) provided greatest resistance to inversion. Metcalfe et al (1997) compared zinc oxide closed basketweave with heel locks and figure-of-eight, reinforced with moleskin tape to a Swede-O-Universal brace, and found no differences between the three methods in terms of talocrural and subtalar range of motion.

Of course, neither ankle taping nor bracing can be regarded as helpful if an athlete's sports performance is affected. A systematic review and meta-analysis of 17 randomized controlled trials (Cordova et al 2005) analysed the effect of ankle taping and bracing on performance. They calculated that there was a performance decrease in sprint speed (1%), agility speed (1%) and vertical jump (0.5%); the worst effect was from a lace-up style brace. Although these figures seem reassuringly trivial, two questions remain: will such small decreases affect the performance of sports people at the elite level? Do the benefits of preventing ankle injury outweigh the small risks of detriment to performance?

PATELLAR TAPING

The investigations into the relationship between mechanical and functional aspects of ankle taping are paralleled over the years by those on patellar taping. It is well known that McConnell (1986) originally described patellar taping as part of an overall treatment programme for patellofemoral pain syndrome (PFPS) and theorized that this technique could alter patellar position, enhance contraction of the vastus medialis oblique (VMO) muscle, and hence decrease pain.

It is becoming clear from recent literature reviews on this subject (Callaghan 1997, Crossley et al 2000) that studies thus far on patients with PFPS have been inconclusive regarding patellar taping enhancement of VMO contractions and taping realignment of patellar position. Nevertheless, there are several studies assessing taping's effect on chronic patellofemoral pain, summarized in a systematic review and meta-analysis (Warden et al 2007). Combined analysis of 13 eligible trials showed that medially directed taping decreased chronic non-arthritic patellar pain immediately and significantly when compared to placebo tape and no tape. The placebo effect probably accounted for 50% of the pain reduction.

More recently, there has been speculation that there is a more subtle role for patellar taping in providing sensory feedback, thereby influencing the proprioceptive status and neuromuscular control of the patellofemoral joint. For example, Callaghan et al (2002) showed that a simple application of one 10-cm strip of patellar taping significantly improved the knee proprioceptive status of healthy subjects whose proprioception was graded as 'poor'. At the same time, Baker et al (2002) showed that patients with PFPS had worse proprioception compared to a group of healthy subjects. Callaghan et al (2008) developed these findings further and measured an improvement in proprioception of PFPS patients by applying non-directional patellar tape. It is tempting therefore to speculate that patellar taping enhances proprioception in patients with patellofemoral pain, and this may explain the short-term subjective improvement without any firm evidence of patellar realignment or VMO-enhanced contractions.

REFERENCES

Alt W, Lohrer H, Gollhofer A 1999 Functional properties of adhesive ankle taping: neuromuscular and mechanical effects before and after exercise. Foot and Ankle International 20(4):238–245

Ashton-Miller JA, Ottaviani RA, Hutchinson C et al 1996 What best protects the inverted weight bearing ankle against further inversion. American Journal of Sports Medicine 24(6):800–809

Bahr R 2001 Recent advances. Sports medicine. British Medical Journal 323:328–331

Baker V, Bennell K, Stillman B et al 2002 Abnormal knee joint position sense in individuals with patellofemoral pain syndrome. Journal of Orthopaedic Research 20:208–214

Callaghan MJ 1997 Patellar taping, the theory versus the evidence: a review. Physical Therapy Reviews 2:181–183

Callaghan MJ, Selfe J, Bagley P et al 2002 The effect of patellar taping on knee joint proprioception. Journal of Athletic Training 37(1):19–24

Callaghan MJ, Selfe J, McHenry A et al 2008 Effects of patellar taping on knee joint proprioception in patients with patellofemoral pain syndrome. Manual Therapy 13:192–199

Cordova ML, Scott BD, Ingersoll CD et al 2005 Effects of ankle support on lower-extremity functional performance: a meta-analysis. Medicine and Science in Sport and Exercise 37(4):635–641

Crossley K, Cowan SM, Bennell KL et al 2000 Patellar taping: is clinical success supported by scientific evidence? Manual Therapy 5(3):142–150

Feuerbach JW, Grabiner MD, Koh TJ et al 1994 Effect of an ankle orthosis and ankle ligament anesthesia on ankle joint proprioception. American Journal of Sports Medicine 22(2):223–229

Frankeny JR, Jewett DL, Hanks GA et al 1993 A comparison of ankle taping methods. Clinical Journal of Sport Medicine 3:20–25

Freeman MAR, Dean MRE, Hanham IWF 1965 The etiology and prevention of functional instability of the foot. Journal of Bone and Joint Surgery (Br) 47-B(4):678–685

Garrick JG, Requa RK 1973 Role of external support in the prevention of ankle sprains. Medicine and Science in Sports 5(3):200–203

Glick JM, Gordon RM, Nishimoto D 1976 The prevention and treatment of ankle injuries. American Journal of Sports Medicine 4:136–141

Greene TA, Hillman SK 1990 Comparison of support provided by a semirigid orthosis and adhesive ankle taping before, during and after exercise. American Journal of Sports Medicine 18(5):498–506

Hamill J, Knutzen KM, Bates BT et al 1986 Evaluation of two ankle appliances using ground reaction force data. Journal of Orthopaedic and Sports Physical Therapy 7(5): 244–249

Handoll H, Rowe B, Quinn KM et al 2001 Interventions for preventing ankle ligament injuries. Cochrane Database of Systematic Reviews, Issue 3. Art. No.: CD000018. DOI: 10.1002/14651858.CD000018

Jerosch J, Hoffstetter I, Bork H et al 1995 The influence of orthoses on the proprioception of the ankle joint. Knee Surgery, Sports Traumatology, Arthroscopy 3:39–46

Karlsson J, Andreasson GO 1992 The effect of external ankle support in chronic lateral ankle joint instability. American Journal of Sports Medicine 20(3):257–261

Kerkhoffs GM, Rowe BH, Assendelft WJ et al 2002a Immobilisation and functional treatment for acute lateral ankle ligament injuries in adults. Cochrane Database of Systematic Reviews 2002, Issue 3. Art. No.: CD003762. DOI: 10.1002/14651858.CD003762

Kerkhoffs GM, Struijs PA, Marti RK et al 2002b Different functional treatment strategies for acute lateral ankle ligament injuries in adults. Cochrane Database of Systematic Reviews 2002, Issue 3. Art. No.: CD002938. DOI: 10.1002/14651858.CD002938

Konradsen L, Hojsgaard C 1993 Pre-heel-strike peroneal muscle activity during walking and running with and without an external ankle support. Scandinavian Journal of Medicine and Science in Sports 3:99–103

Konradsen L, Ravn J, Sorensen AI 1993 Proprioception at the ankle: the effect of anaesthetic blockade of ligament receptors. Journal of Bone and Joint Surgery (Br) 75-B(3):433–436

Konradsen L, Beynnon BD, Renström PA 2000 Techniques for measuring sensorimotor control of the ankle: evaluation of different methods. In: Lephart SM, Fu FH (eds) Proprioception and neuromuscular control in joint stability, 1st edn. Human Kinetics, Champaign, pp 139–144

Larsen E 1984 Taping the ankle for chronic instability. Acta Orthopaedica Scandinavica 55:551–553

Laughman RK, Carr TA, Chao E et al 1980 Three dimensional kinematics of the taped ankle before and after exercise. American Journal of Sports Medicine 8(6):425–431

Lentell G, Baas B, Lopez D et al 1995 The contributions of proprioceptive deficits, muscle function, and anatomic laxity to functional instability of the ankle. Journal of Orthopaedic and Sports Physical Therapy 21(4):206–215

Lohrer H, Alt W, Gollhofer A 1999 Neuromuscular properties and functional aspects of taped ankles. American Journal of Sports Medicine 27(1):69–75

McCluskey GM, Blackburn TA, Lewis T 1976 A treatment for ankle sprains. American Journal of Sports Medicine 4(4):158–161

McConnell J 1986 The management of chondromalacia patellae: a long term solution. Australian Journal of Physiotherapy 32(4):215–223

Manfroy PP, Ashton-Miller JA, Wojtys EM 1997 The effect of exercise, prewrap and athletic tape on the maximal active and passive ankle resistance to ankle inversion. American Journal of Sports Medicine 25(2):156–163

Meana M, Alegre LM, Elvira JL et al 2007 Kinematics of ankle taping after a training session. International Journal of Sports Medicine 29(1):70–76

Metcalfe RC, Schlabach GA, Looney MA et al 1997 A comparison of moleskin tape, linen tape and lace up brace on joint restriction and movement performance. Journal of Athletic Training 32(2):136–140

Myburgh KH, Vaughan CL, Issacs SK 1984 The effects of ankle guards and taping on joint motion before, during and after a squash match. American Journal of Sports Medicine 12(6):441–446

Rarick GL, Bigley G, Karts R et al 1962 The measurable support of the ankle joint by conventional methods of taping. Journal of Bone and Joint Surgery (Am) 44(A6):1183–1190

Refshauge KM, Kilbreath SL, Raymond J 2000 The effect of recurrent ankle inversion sprain and taping on proprioception at the ankle. Medicine and Science in Sport and Exercise 32(1):10–15

Ricard MD, Sherwood SM, Schulthies SS et al 2000 Effects of tape and exercise on dynamic ankle inversion. Journal of Athletic Training 35(1):31–37

Robbins S, Waked E, Rappel R 1995 Ankle taping improves proprioception before and after exercise in young men. British Journal of Sports Medicine 29(4):242–247

Rucinski TJ, Hooker DN, Prentice WE et al 1991 The effects of intermittent compression on edema in postacute ankle sprains. Journal of Orthopaedic and Sports Physical Therapy 14(2):65–69

Sharpe SR, Knapik J, Jones B 1997 Ankle braces effectively reduce recurrence of ankle sprains in female soccer players. Journal of Athletic Training 32(1):21–24

Sitler M, Ryan J, Wheeler B et al 1994 The efficacy of a semirigid ankle stabilizer to reduce acute ankle injuries in basketball. A randomized clinical study at West Point. American Journal of Sports Medicine 22(4):454–461

Spanos S, Brunswic M, Billis E 2008 The effect of taping on the proprioception of the ankle in a non-weight bearing position, amongst injured athletes. The Foot 18(1):25–33

Surve I, Schwellnus MP, Noakes T et al 1994 A five-fold reduction in the incidence of recurrent ankle sprains in soccer players using the sport-stirrup orthosis. American Journal of Sports Medicine 22(5):601–605

Tropp H, Askling C, Gillquist J 1985 Prevention of ankle sprains. American Journal of Sports Medicine 13(4):259–262

Vaes P, DeBoeck H, Handelberg F et al 1985 Comparative radiological study of the influence of ankle joint strapping and taping on ankle stability. Journal of Orthopaedic and Sports Physical Therapy 7(3):110–114

Viljakka T 1986 Mechanics of knee and ankle bandages. Acta Orthopaedica Scandinavica 57:54–58

Warden SJ, Hinman RS, Watson MA Jr et al 2007 Patellar taping and bracing for the treatment of chronic knee pain: A systematic review and meta-analysis. Arthritis and Rheumatism 59(1):73–83

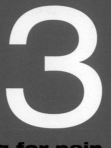

3

chapter
◄◄

Taping for pain relief

J. McConnell

CHAPTER CONTENTS

Pain is the most frequent complaint of patients presenting for treatment at sports medicine clinics. However, pain is usually not the result of an acute one-off injury but of habitual imbalances in the movement system which over time cause chronic problems. The management of musculoskeletal symptoms is therefore extremely challenging for the clinician, as symptom reduction alone is not sufficient for a successful treatment outcome, particularly when dealing with athletes who need to be finely tuned for the extraordinary demands placed on their bodies. Often it is difficult for the clinician to determine the cause and origin of the pain as there may be confounding hyper/hypomobility problems of the surrounding soft tissues. One of the greatest challenges for a patient is finding appropriate strategies to stabilize any unstable segments, as success in this area will ensure fewer recurrences and perhaps a higher return of function.

Joint stability requires the interaction of three different subsystems – the passive (the bones, ligaments, fascia and any other non-contractile tissue such as discs and menisci), the active (the muscles acting on the joints) and the neural (central nervous system and nerves controlling the muscles) subsystems (Panjabi 1992a). The most vulnerable area of a joint is known as the neutral zone, where little resistance is offered by the passive structures (Panjabi 1992b). Dysfunction of the passive, active or neural systems will affect the neutral zone and hence the stability of the joint. The size of the neutral zone can be increased by injury and decreased with muscle strengthening. In the spine, for example, stability of a segment can be increased by muscle activity of as little as 1–3% (Cholewicki et al 1997). Uncompensated dysfunction, however, will ultimately cause pathology.

How long will it take before uncompensated movement causes symptoms? The answer to this question is probably best determined by Dye's model of tissue homeostasis of a joint (Dye 1996). Dye contends that symptoms will only occur when an individual is no longer operating inside his/her envelope of function, reaching a particular threshold and thereby causing a complex biological cascade of trauma and repair, manifesting clinically as pain and swelling. The threshold varies from individual to individual, depending on the amount and frequency of the loading (Dye 1996, Novacheck 1997). Four factors (anatomic, kinematic, physiological and treatment) are pertinent in determining the size of the envelope of function (Dye 1996, Dye et al 1998). The therapist can have a positive influence on the patient's envelope of function by minimizing the aggravation of the inflamed tissue and can perhaps even increase the patient's threshold of function by improving the control over the mobile segments and the movement of the stiff segments (McConnell 2000).

MINIMIZING THE AGGRAVATION OF INFLAMED TISSUE – UNLOADING PAINFUL STRUCTURES

The concept of minimizing the aggravation of inflamed tissue is certainly central to all interventions in orthopaedics. Clinicians have a number of weapons in their armoury, such as anti-inflammatory medication, topical creams, ice, electrotherapy modalities, acupuncture and tape, to attack pain and reduce inflammation. It is in the chronic state that pain is more difficult to settle and sometimes symptoms seem to be increased by the very treatment that is designed to diminish them. For example, a patient with chronic low-back and leg pain with restricted forward flexion, treated in slump to increase range, experiences a marked exacerbation of the symptoms. This patient becomes reluctant to have further treatment for fear of further increase in pain; thus, the range becomes more restricted, further reducing the patient's activity. Another patient, with chronic fat pad irritation, is given straight-leg-raise exercises, only to find the pain worsens, so avoids further treatment and limits activity, which hastens the quadriceps atrophy, resulting in lateral tracking of the patella and further increases in pain. The infrapatellar fat pad is one of the most pain-sensitive structures in the knee and must be respected as a potent source of anterior knee symptoms (Dye et al 1998).

Key to the success of management of these patients is to unload the inflamed soft tissues to break the endless cycle of increased pain and decreased activity, which allows the clinician to address the patient's poor dynamic control. The principle of unloading is based on the premise that inflamed soft tissue does not respond well to stretch (Gresalmer & McConnell 1998). For example, if a patient presents with a sprained medial collateral ligament, applying a valgus stress to the knee will aggravate the condition, whereas a varus stress will decrease the symptoms. Tape can be used to unload (shorten) the inflamed tissue and perhaps improve joint alignment by providing a constant low load on the soft tissue. It has been widely documented that the length of soft tissues can be increased with sustained stretching (Herbert 1993, Hooley et al 1980). If the tape can be maintained for a prolonged period of time, then this, plus muscle training of the stabilizing muscles actively to change the joint position, be it patellofemoral (PF) or glenohumeral, should have a significant effect on the mechanics.

There is some debate as to whether tape can actually change joint position. Most of the research has examined changes in patellar position. Some investigators have found that tape changes PF angle and lateral patellar displacement, but congruence angle is not changed (Roberts 1989). Others have concurred, finding no change in congruence angle when the patella is taped, but congruence angle is measured at 45° knee flexion, so subtle changes in patellar position may have occurred before this (Bockrath et al 1993). A recent study of asymptomatic subjects found that medial glide tape was effective in moving the patella medially (P = 0.003), but ineffective in maintaining the position after vigorous exercise (P < 0.001). But tape seemed to prevent the lateral shift of the patella that occurred with exercise (P = 0.016) (Larsen et al 1995). The issue for a therapist, however, is not whether the tape changes the patellar position on X-ray, but whether the therapist can immediately decrease the patient's symptoms by at least 50%, so the patient can exercise and train in a pain-free manner.

EFFECT OF TAPE

The effect of tape on pain, particularly PF pain, has been fairly well established in the literature (Bockrath et al 1993, Cerny 1995, Conway et al 1992, Gilleard et al 1998, Powers et al 1997). Even in an older age group (mean age 70 years) with tibiofemoral osteoarthritis, taping the patella in a medial direction resulted in a 25% reduction in knee pain (Cushnagan et al 1994). However, the mechanism of the effect is still widely debated.

It has been found that taping the patella of symptomatic individuals such that the pain is decreased by 50% results in an earlier activation of the vastus medialis oblique (VMO) relative to the vastus lateralis (VL) on ascending and descending stairs. The VMO during stair descent activated 8.3° earlier than the VL in the taped condition, as taping the patella not only resulted in an earlier activation of the VMO but a significantly delayed activation of the VL (Gilleard et al 1998). This result has recently been confirmed by Cowan et al (2002), where it was found that tape leads to a change in the onset timing of the VMO relative to the VL compared with placebo tape and no tape.

Patellar taping has also been associated with increases in loading response knee flexion, as well as increases in quadriceps muscle torque (Conway et al 1992, Handfield & Kramer 2000, Powers et al 1997). When the quadriceps torque of symptomatic army personnel was evaluated in taped, braced and control conditions, it was found that the taped group generated both higher concentric and eccentric torque than both the control and braced groups. There was, however, no correlation between the increase in muscle torque and the amount of pain reduction (Conway et al 1992).

It has been suggested that patellar tape could influence the magnitude of VMO and VL activation but the results of a limited number of studies have not supported this contention (Cerny 1995).

PATELLAR TAPING

Patellar taping is unique to each patient, as the components corrected, the order of correction and the tension of the tape are tailored for each individual based on the assessment of the patellar position. The worst component is always corrected first and the effect of each piece of tape on the patient's symptoms should be evaluated by reassessing the painful activity. It may be necessary to correct more than one component. After each piece of tape is applied, the symptom-producing activity should be reassessed. If the tape does not change the patient's symptoms immediately or even worsens them, one of the following must be considered:

- the patient requires tape to unload the soft tissues
- the tape was poorly applied
- the assessment of patellar position was inadequate
- the patient has an intra-articular primary pathology which was inappropriate for taping.

If a posterior tilt problem has been ascertained on assessment, it must be corrected first, as taping over the inferior pole of the patella will aggravate the fat pad and exacerbate the patient's pain. With acute fat pad irritation, the pain is exacerbated by extension manoeuvres such as straight-leg raises and prolonged standing (McConnell 1991). Therefore any treatment that involves quadriceps setting will exacerbate the symptoms.

UNLOADING NEURAL TISSUE – A STRATEGY FOR MANAGING CHRONIC LOW-BACK AND LEG PAIN

Tape may be used to unload inflamed neural tissue. The unloading tape enables the patient to be treated without an increase in symptoms, so that, in the long term, treatment is more efficacious. The mechanism of the effect is yet to be investigated, but tape could:

- inhibit an overactive hamstring muscle, which is a protective response to mechanical provocation of neural tissue
- have some effect on changing the orientation of the fascia
- have just a proprioceptive effect, working on the pain gate mechanism (Jerosch et al 1996, Verhagen et al 2000).

The tape is applied along the affected dermatome region such that the soft tissue is lifted up towards the spine. The buttock is always unloaded (Fig. 3.1), starting medial in the gluteal fold, taping proximal to the greater trochanter while lifting the soft tissue up towards the iliac crest. This is followed by a tape which is parallel to the natal cleft, ending at the posterior superior iliac spine (PSIS), and a third tape joining the first two tapes from

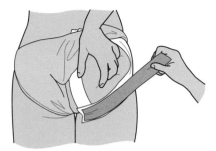

Figure 3.1 Unloading the buttock to decrease leg symptoms. The tape must be sculptured into the gluteal fold.

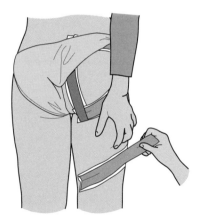

Figure 3.2 For S1 distribution of pain, the posterior thigh is taped, with the skin being lifted to the buttock. If the proximal symptoms worsen, the tape diagonal should be reversed.

lateral to medial. A diagonal strip is placed halfway down the thigh over the appropriate dermatome and the soft tissue is lifted towards the spine (for S1 dermatome, see Fig. 3.2).

The direction of the tape depends on symptom reduction. The symptoms above the tape should be reduced immediately; the distal symptoms, however, may be exacerbated. If the proximal symptoms are worsened, the tape direction should be changed immediately (if worse, reverse), which should have the effect of improving the symptoms. Distal symptoms will be improved when a diagonal strip is placed midway down on the

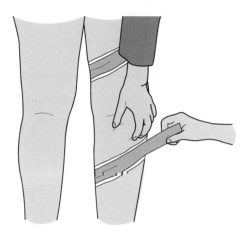

Figure 3.3 Unloading the calf to decrease S1 symptoms.

lower leg over the symptomatic dermatome and the soft tissue is lifted proximally (Fig. 3.3). Once the tissues are unloaded the patient can be treated without an increase in symptoms.

When managing low-back and leg pain, the clinician may need to change the treatment focus, so that the treatment is not just directed at the involved segment but addresses the contributory factors. Patients with chronic back and leg pain often have internally rotated femurs; this reduces the available hip extension and external rotation range, causing an increase in the rotation in the lumbar spine when the patient walks. The internal rotation in the hip also causes tightness in the iliotibial band and diminished activity in the gluteus medius posterior fibres, so the pelvis exhibits dynamic instability. The lack of control around the pelvis further increases the movement of an already mobile lumbar spine segment. It has been established that excessive movement, particularly in rotation, is a contributory factor to disc injury and the torsional forces may irrevocably damage fibres of the annulus fibrosis (Farfan et al 1970, Kelsey et al 1984). Therefore, an excessive amount of movement about the lumbar spine because of limited hip movement and control, in combination with poor abdominal support, may be a significant factor in the development of low-back pain.

Treatment of chronic low-back pain should be directed at:

- increasing hip and thoracic spine mobility to ensure a more even distribution of the motion through the body for functional activities
- improving the stability, rather than mobility, of the relevant lumbar segments. This involves muscle control of the multifidus, transversus

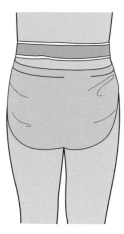

Figure 3.4 Stabilizing an unstable lumbar segment.

abdominis (TA) and the posterior fibres of the gluteus medius. As it can take a considerable period of time for specific muscle training to be effective, tape can be used to help stabilize the vulnerable lumbar segments while the muscles are being trained (Fig. 3.4).

SHOULDER TAPING – REPOSITIONING OR UNLOADING

The shoulder, like the PF joint, is a soft-tissue joint whereby its position is controlled by the soft tissues around it. Poor muscle function, particularly around the scapula, and stiffness in the thoracic spine will severely affect shoulder function, making it susceptible to instability and impingement problems. In fact, most shoulder pathology relates to these two factors in some way. Impingement causes mechanical irritation of the rotator cuff tendons, resulting in haemorrhage and swelling, usually as a result of:

- encroachment from above – either congenital abnormalities or osteophyte formation
- swelling of the rotator cuff tendons – usually an overuse tendinitis associated with poor biomechanics, such as a faulty throwing or swimming technique
- excessive translation of the humeral head. Chronic anterior instability results in increased translation of the humeral head in an anterosuperior direction narrowing the subacromial space. Laxity of the anterior shoulder develops over time due to repeated stressing of the static stabilizers at the extremes of motion, for example the cocking motion in pitchers.

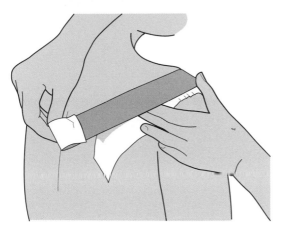

Figure 3.5 Tape to reposition the humeral head, decreasing the forward translation of the humeral head.

It is possible to increase the space available for the soft-tissue structures by repositioning the humeral head (Fig. 3.5).

The aim of the tape is to lift the anterior aspect of the humeral head up and back so that there is increased space between the acromion and the elevating humerus. The tape is anchored over the inferior border of the scapula. Care must be taken not to pull too hard anteriorly, as the skin is sensitive in this region and will break down if not looked after properly. The tape can remain in situ for about a week, depending on symptom reduction. Improving thoracic spine mobility and muscle training of the scapular and glenohumeral stabilizers must be addressed in treatment to ensure long-term reduction in symptoms. Athletic individuals with shoulder problems often have extremely poor trunk and pelvic stabilization, which also needs to be addressed in treatment to improve their athletic performance.

CONCLUSION

Musculoskeletal pain can be difficult to treat as the clinician not only has to identify the underlying causative factors to restore homeostasis to the system, but also has to ensure that the treatment does not unnecessarily exacerbate the symptoms. In some cases the clinician may need to unload the painful structures before commencing any other intervention. Tape can be used successfully to achieve this aim. Tape not only unloads painful tissue but it can facilitate underactive muscles as well as inhibit excessive muscle activity. The therapist receives immediate feedback from the patient as to whether the tape application has been successful or not. Tape can be adapted to suit the individual patient. It is readily adjusted and the tension can be varied. Tape is relatively cost-effective and time-efficient, so the therapist should be innovative and creative if symptom reduction has not been achieved, as tape can facilitate treatment outcome.

REFERENCES

Bockrath K, Wooden C, Worrell T et al 1993 Effects of patella taping on patella position and perceived pain. Medicine Science in Sports and Exercise 25(9):989–992

Cerny K 1995 Vastus medialis oblique/vastus lateralis muscle activity ratios for selected exercises in persons with and without patellofemoral pain syndrome. Physical Therapy 75(8):672–683

Cholewicki J, Panjabi MM, Khachatryan A 1997 Stabilizing function of trunk flexor-extensor muscles around a neutral spine posture. Spine 22(19):2207–2212

Conway A, Malone T, Conway P 1992 Patellar alignment/tracking alteration: effect on force output and perceived pain. Isokinetics and Exercise Science 2(1):9–17

Cowan SM, Bennell KL, Crossley KM et al 2002 Physical therapy alters recruitment of the vasti in patellofemoral pain syndrome. Medicine and Science in Sports and Exercise 34(12):1879–1885

Cushnaghan J, McCarthy R, Dieppe P 1994 The effect of taping the patella on pain in the osteoarthritic patient. British Medical Journal 308:753–755

Dye S 1996 The knee as a biologic transmission with an envelope of function: a theory. Clinical Orthopaedics 325:10–18

Dye S, Vaupel G, Dye C 1998 Conscious neurosensory mapping of the internal structures of the human knee without intra-articular anaesthesia. American Journal of Sports Medicine 26(6):1–5

Farfan HF, Cossette JW, Robertson GH et al 1970 The effects of torsion on lumbar intervertebral joints: the role of torsion in the production of disc degeneration. Journal of Bone and Joint Surgery 52A:468–497

Gilleard W, McConnell J, Parsons D 1998 The effect of patellar taping on the onset of vastus medialis obliquus and vastus lateralis muscle activity in persons with patellofemoral pain. Physical Therapy 78(1):25–32

Gresalmer R, McConnell J 1998 The patella: a team approach. Aspen, Gaithersburg, MD

Handfield T, Kramer J 2000 Effect of McConnell taping on perceived pain and knee extensor torques during isokinetic exercise performed by patients with patellofemoral pain syndrome. Physiotherapy Canada (winter):39–44

Herbert R 1993 Preventing and treating stiff joints. In: Crosbie J, McConnell J (eds) Key issues in musculoskeletal physiotherapy. Butterworth-Heinemann, Oxford

Hooley C, McCrum N, Cohen R 1980 The visco-elastic deformation of the tendon. Journal of Biomechanics 13:521

Jerosch J, Thorwesten L, Bork H 1996 Is prophylactic bracing of the ankle cost effective? Orthopedics 19(5):405–414

Kelsey JL, Githens PB, White AA 1984 An epidemiological study of lifting and twisting on the job and the risk for acute prolapsed lumbar intervertebral disc. Journal of Orthopaedic Research 2:61–66

Larsen B, Andreasen E, Urfer A et al 1995 Patellar taping: a radiographic examination of the medial glide technique. American Journal of Sports Medicine 23:465–471

McConnell J 1991 Fat pad irritation – a mistaken patellar tendonitis. Sport Health 9(4):7–9

McConnell J 2000 A novel approach to pain relief pre-therapeutic exercise. Journal of Science Medicine and Sport 3(3):325–334

Novacheck TF 1997 The biomechanics of running and sprinting. In: Guten GN (ed.) Running injuries. WB Saunders, Philadelphia, PA, pp 4–19

Panjabi M 1992a The stabilising system of the spine. Part I. Function dysfunction adaptation and enhancement. Journal of Spinal Disorders 5(4):383–389

Panjabi M 1992b The stabilising system of the spine. Part II. Neutral zone and instability hypothesis. Journal of Spinal Disorders 5(4):390–397

Powers C, Landel R, Sosnick T et al 1997 The effects of patellar taping on stride characteristics and joint motion in subjects with patellofemoral pain. Journal of Orthopaedic Sports and Physical Therapy 26(6):286–291

Roberts JM 1989 The effect of taping on patellofemoral alignment – a radiological pilot study. In: Proceedings of the Sixth Biennial Conference of the Manipulative Therapists Association of Australia, pp 146–151

Verhagen EA, van Mechelen W, de Vente W 2000 The effect of preventive measures on the incidence of ankle sprains. Clinical Journal of Sport Medicine 10(4):291–296

4

chapter

◄◄|

Recent taping techniques to alter muscle activity and proprioception

U. McCarthy Persson

CHAPTER CONTENTS

INTRODUCTION

The use of tape in the management, prevention and treatment of neuro-musculoskeletal injuries has become common practice. Recently, taping techniques with the primary purpose of altering muscle activity have become common physiotherapy treatment options. There is a small but growing base of scientific evidence for some of these taping applications.

This chapter examines the evidence in the current literature of taping techniques with the primary purpose of altering muscle activity.

SHOULDER TAPE

Patients with scapulothoracic dysfunction have a tendency to have hypertrophy or hyperactivity of the upper trapezius muscle in relation to the middle and lower portions (Morin et al 1997).

Inhibitory upper trapezius tape

Tape applied firmly across the fibres of a muscle has been proposed to decrease the activity of a muscle (Morrissey 2000). A number of studies have tested this hypothesis, mainly by applying rigid tape firmly, perpendicular to the direction of the muscle fibres over the upper trapezius (Fig. 4.1) and the vastus lateralis muscles (See Fig. 4.2) (Cools et al 2002, Janwantankul & Gaogasigam 2005, Morin et al 1997, Selkowitz et al 2007, Tobin & Robinson 2000).

A study using an isometric muscle contraction of the upper trapezius into scapular retraction and elevation showed that the effects of the

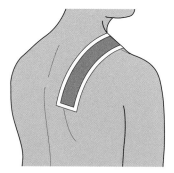

Figure 4.1 Inhibitory upper trapezius tape (Morrissey 2000).

upper trapezius inhibitory taping resulted in a significant decrease in electromyographic (EMG) activity of the upper trapezius muscle and an increase in EMG activity in the middle portion of the trapezius muscle while taped when compared with a no-tape condition (Morin et al 1997).

Another study using a different methodology examined the EMG activity of the scapular muscles during active shoulder flexion and abduction (Cools et al 2002) and failed to find any significant changes in EMG activity of the upper and lower trapezius or the serratus anterior with similar inhibitory tape applied. Only one study has examined the effects of the upper trapezius inhibitory tape in subjects with shoulder pain (Selkowitz et al 2007). The results from this study indicate that this taping technique can inhibit the upper trapezius with a resulting increase in activity in the lower trapezius muscle during shoulder elevation when compared to an untaped condition.

The differences in methodology of these three studies make it difficult to draw conclusions about the absolute effects of inhibitory taping over the upper trapezius. Present evidence indicates that a single strip of rigid tape may decrease upper trapezius muscle activity and increase activity of the middle/lower trapezius during isometric contraction and shoulder elevation in patients with shoulder pain.

Tape to facilitate the scapular muscles

One study examined the effects of a taping technique intended to increase a specific muscle's activity. This study assessed a muscle's readiness to contract using the H-reflex (Alexander et al 2003). The H-reflex can be seen as an electrically evoked equivalent of the tendon jerk reflex and gives an indication of the amount of motor unit activation available in a particular muscle (Schieppati 1987). In the study, a tape was applied across the scapula towards the spine in a fashion believed to facilitate the underlying muscle with tension applied on the tape in the line of the lower trapezius muscle fibres, as previously suggested by Morrissey (2000). Contrary to the authors' expectations, the H-reflex was decreased by the tape indicating an inhibition rather than a facilitation of the lower trapezius muscle (Alexander et al 2003).

Proprioceptive taping

Two studies attempted to assess the effect of tape on proprioception and performance in the shoulder.

The ability to reposition the scapula during active shoulder flexion and abduction was studied by Zanella et al (2001) with and without a scapular tape. The scapular tape was not found to increase the ability to reposition the scapula in normal subjects or subjects with a 'winging' scapula.

In another study, a scapular tape retracting both scapulae was applied in an attempt to improve scapular position and muscular performance in professional violinists without shoulder pathology. The EMG activity of the trapezii and scapular retractor muscles and the quality of music performance were assessed. Contrary to the authors' expectations, when compared to a no-tape control condition, the tape significantly increased the EMG activity of the upper trapezius muscle and there was a decrease in quality of the music performance (Ackermann et al 2002).

INHIBITORY VASTUS LATERALIS TAPE

The patellofemoral joint has been described as the most researched small joint in the body, producing pain and disability far out of proportion to its shape and size (Gerrard 1995). One of the underlying theories behind the cause of patellofemoral pain syndrome (PFPS) is that there is an imbalance between the contraction of vastus lateralis (VL) and vastus medialis obliquus (VMO) muscles (McConnell 1986).

Patella taping is a common technique used for patients with PFPS and aims to realign the patella and increase the activity of the VMO (McConnell 1996). Another approach is to attempt to decrease the muscle activity of the VL and thereby address patellar pathomechanics (Tobin & Robinson 2000).

There are currently only two studies published on inhibitory taping of the VL and its effect on muscle activity, both studies investigating surface EMG during stair *descent* (Janwantankul & Gaogasigam 2005, Tobin & Robinson 2000). Stair *walking* has been described as one of the most challenging and pain-provoking activities in individuals with PFPS (Gilleard et al 1998). Tobin & Robinson (2000) applied the tape perpendicular to the fibres of the VL muscle with enough tension to form a furrow in the skin (Fig. 4.2). Electromyographic data were collected from the VMO and the VL muscles. The authors reported a significant decrease in EMG activity of the VL while the VMO remained unchanged. However, there are some concerns raised about the methodology of this study in that the pace of stair walking was not controlled and the EMG data were sampled at very low frequency (Herrington 2000, Scott 2000).

Janwantankul & Gaogasigam (2005) attempted to repeat and improve the methodology of Tobin & Robinson (2000). The authors assessed mean EMG activity during stair *descent* with tape applied perpendicular to the VL muscle fibres but also parallel to the muscle fibres, aiming to facilitate muscle activity (Morrissey 2000). There was no significant difference in the EMG activity of the VMO and VL compared with the no-tape condition. Unfortunately elastic tape was used rather than the rigid tape which has been used in all other similar studies assessing inhibitory tape techniques.

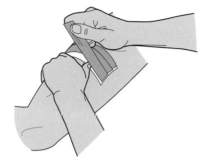

Figure 4.2 Vastus lateralis inhibitory tape applied firmly, perpendicular to the muscle fibres.

These two studies differ to such an extent that it is difficult to draw direct comparisons and identify how this type of inhibitory tape affects the muscle activity.

To achieve a greater understanding of the effects of the VL inhibitory tape, a repeatable application procedure has been established (McCarthy Persson et al 2007a) and the effects during stair *ascent* and *descent* assessed (McCarthy Persson et al 2008). The results from this study concur with Tobin & Robinson's (2000) results that a selective inhibition of the VL can occur during stair *descent* but also during *ascent*.

Two studies have assessed the effects of tape applied to increase or decrease the muscle activity of the calf muscle (Alexander et al 2008, McCarthy Persson et al 2007b). Both these studies used the H-reflex to assess the effects of the tape applications on the muscle. While McCarthy Persson et al (2007b) noted an increase in the soleus H-reflex, Alexander et al (2008) found no such change in the H-reflex with the tape applied perpendicular to the muscle fibres. The latter study found that application of a rigid tape parallel to the muscle fibre decreased the H-reflex of the medial gastrocnemius muscle (Alexander et al 2008). These results are again conflicting, and the tape application varies with a greater reported tension application in the McCarthy Persson (2007b) study, and a different angulation of the tape.

PROPOSED MECHANISM OF ACTION

From the published literature there is some evidence that rigid tape applied across the muscle fibres of the upper trapezius and VL can inhibit the muscle activity during functional movements. There is also evidence that tape applied parallel to the muscle fibres of the lower trapezius and medial gastrocnemius decreases the motor neurone excitability during static conditions.

It has been suggested that the inhibition caused by tape parallel to the muscle fibres may be due to the tape shortening the muscle (Morrissey 2000). If the tape was able to shorten the muscle, it may off-load the muscle spindle and thereby decrease its tonic discharge and reduce the H-reflex (Alexander et al 2008).

Other proposed mechanisms have been suggested such as alterations in muscle activity from the tape causing mechanoreceptor stimulation in the skin. It has been found that the mechanoreceptor activation is dependent on the direction of tension applied to the skin (Olausson et al 2000). It has furthermore been demonstrated that application of tension on the skin in a particular direction will cause a particular change in muscle activity (MacGregor et al 2005). It was found that when tape was applied with tension over the patella in subjects with PFPS, a selective increase in activity of the VMO occurred. This increase in muscle activity was greatest when the skin was stretched in a lateral direction (MacGregor et al 2005). Research involving these relatively new taping techniques is still scarce. There is need for further exploration of the effects and mechanisms of actions underlying taping techniques to alter muscle activity and proprioception.

REFERENCES

Ackermann B, Adams R, Marshall E 2002 The effect of scapula taping on electromyographic activity and musical performance in professional violinists. Australian Journal of Physiotherapy 48:197–204

Alexander CM, Stynes S, Thomas A et al 2003 Does tape facilitate or inhibit the lower trapezius? Manual Therapy 8(1):37–41

Alexander MA, McMullan M, Harrison PJ 2008 What is the effect of taping along or across a muscle on a motorneurone excitability? A study using the triceps surae. Manual Therapy 13:57–62

Cools AM, Witvrouw EE, Dannieels LA et al 2002 Does taping influence electromyographic muscle activity in the scapular rotators in healthy shoulders? Manual Therapy 7(3):154–162

Gerrard B 1995 The patellofemoral complex. In: Zuluaga M (ed.) Sports physiotherapy. Churchill Livingstone, Melbourne, pp 587–611

Gilleard W, McConnell J, Parsons D 1998 The effect of patellar taping on the onset of vastus medialis oblique and vastus lateralis muscle activity in persons with patellofemoral pain. Physical Therapy 78:25–32

Herrington L 2000 Electromyographic problems. Physiotherapy 86(7):390–392

Janwantankul P, Gaogasigam C 2005 Vastus lateralis and vastus medialis obliquus muscle activity during the application of inhibition and facilitation taping techniques. Clinical Rehabilitation 19:12–19

McCarthy Persson JU, Hooper ACB, Fleming HE 2007a Repeatability of skin displacement and pressure during 'inhibitory' vastus lateralis muscle taping. Manual Therapy 12:17–21

McCarthy Persson U, Boland S, Ryan S et al 2007b The effects of an inhibitory muscle tape on the soleus H-reflex. Journal of Orthopaedic and Sports Physical Therapy 37(3): abstract

McCarthy Persson U, Fleming HE, Caulfield B 2008 The effect of a vastus lateralis tape on muscle activity during stair climbing. Man Ther Jul 8 (Epub ahead of print)

McConnell JS 1986 The management of chondromalacia patella: a long term solution. Australian Journal of Physiotherapy 32:215–223

McConnell J 1996 Management of patellofemoral problems. Manual Therapy 1:60–66

MacGregor K, Gerlach S, Mellor S et al 2005 Cutaneus stimulation from patella tape causes a differential increase in vasti muscle activity in people with patellofemoral pain. Journal of Orthopedic Research 23:351–358

Morin GE, Tiberio D, Austin G 1997 The effect of upper trapezius taping on electromyographic activity in the upper and middle trapezius region. Journal of Sport Rehabilitation 6:309–318

Morrissey D 2000 Proprioceptive shoulder taping. Journal of Bodywork and Movement Therapies 4(3):189–194

Olausson H, Wessberg J, Kakuda N 2000 Tactile directional sensibility: peripheral neural mechanisms in man. Brain Research 866(1–2):178–187

Schieppati M 1987 The Hoffmann reflex: a means of assessing spinal reflex excitability and its descending control in man. Progress in Neurobiology 28:345–376

Scott M 2000 Room for improvement in study design. Physiotherapy 86(7):391–392

Selkowitz DM, Chaney C, Stuckey SJ et al 2007 The effects of scapular taping on the surface electromyographic signal amplitude of shoulder girdle muscles during upper extremity elevation in individuals with suspected shoulder impingement syndrome. Journal of Orthopedic and Sports Physical Therapy 37(11):694–702

Tobin S, Robinson G 2000 The effect of vastus lateralis inhibition taping technique on vastus lateralis and vastus medialis obliquus activity. Physiotherapy 86(4):173–183

Zanella PW, Willey SM, Seibel SL et al 2001 The effect of scapular taping on shoulder repositioning. Journal of Sport Rehabilitation 10(2):113–123

part 2

PART CONTENTS

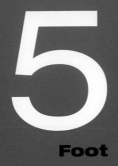

5

chapter

◀◀

Foot

CHAPTER CONTENTS

Turf toe strap

J. O'Neill

INDICATION

First metatarsophalangeal (MTP) joint sprain.

FUNCTION

To stabilize and support the big toe in sprain of the MTP joint.

MATERIALS

Tape adherent, 2.5-cm porous athletic tape, 5-cm light elastic tape.

POSITION

The athlete should be sitting with the foot in a relaxed position over a table.

APPLICATION

1. Apply tape adherent.
2. With the foot and big toe in a neutral position, apply anchor strips to the big toe and midfoot (Fig. 5.1).
3. Apply four to six precut 2.5-cm strips (approximately 15–20 cm long) starting at the big toe and pulling down towards the midfoot anchor, covering completely the MTP joint (dorsal and plantar; Fig. 5.2).
4. Finish by covering the toe with two to three 2.5-cm strips. Cover the midfoot with 5-cm light elastic tape (Fig. 5.3).

CHECK FUNCTION

It is important to check function. The purpose of the tape is to stabilize the joint; if this is not accomplished, pain will result. Therefore the tape must be tightened.

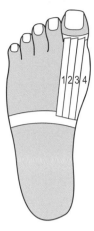

Figure 5.1

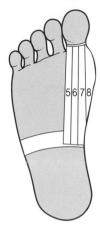

Figure 5.2

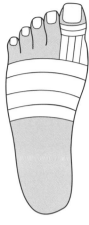

Figure 5.3

Tips

1. If pain is only in one movement of the toes (whether in flexion or extension), prevent only that movement. This allows for greater mobility of the toe.
2. Do not put the toe at an anatomical disadvantage – excessive flexion or extension – to prevent pain.

Hallux valgus

R. Macdonald

INDICATION

Pain in the first MTP joint due to valgus strain.

FUNCTION

To relieve the symptoms and allow walking in comfort. Helps to correct a mild deformity.

MATERIALS

Adhesive spray, 5-cm stretch tape and 2.5-cm rigid tape.

POSITION

Supine, with the foot over the edge of the plinth.

APPLICATION

1. Lightly spray the foot.
2. Using 5-cm stretch tape, attach to the medial side of the proximal phalanx of the great toe, distal to the joint line.
3. Anchor with a strip of 2.5-cm rigid tape around the phalanx to prevent slippage.
4. Draw tape back and around the heel, down the lateral side, under the arch, encircle the midfoot and finish under the arch (Figs 5.4 and 5.5).
5. Close off with a strip of rigid tape.

CHECK FUNCTION

Have the patient walk to check comfort.

CONTRAINDICATION

Ensure the tape is not too tight at the initial stage, as it may cause excessive abduction of the great toe.

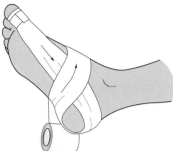

Figure 5.4

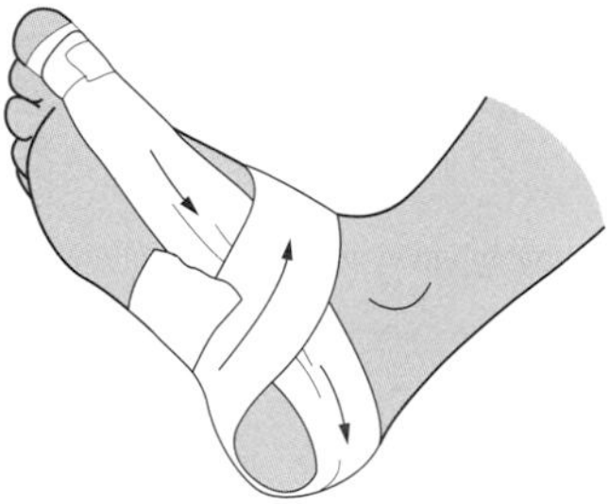

Figure 5.5

Tips

Teach the patient how to apply the technique, as the patient can best judge the amount of abduction for comfort. The abduction may be increased little by little as necessary.

Antipronation taping

A. Hughes

INDICATION

Foot, ankle and lower-limb injuries caused by hyperpronation. A diagnostic tool to assess the value of functional orthotics.

FUNCTION

To limit the degree of calcaneal eversion which occurs early in the stance phase of the gait cycle. To assist plantarflexion of the first ray in late stance phase.

MATERIALS

3.8-cm rigid tape, 5-cm hypoallergenic tape, e.g. Fixomull or Hypafix, for application times that will exceed 4 h.

POSITION

Long sitting with the foot over the end of the bed. Foot/ankle complex maintained in neutral flexion/extension angle.

APPLICATION

Apply the hypoallergenic tape in the same sequence as the rigid tape to follow:

1. Apply two anchors to the forefoot, over and just posterior to the MTP joints, overlapping by two-thirds (Fig. 5.6).
2. The initial support strip is taken with tension from the superomedial anchor back around the calcaneum, and down the lateral side of the calcaneum at an angle of 45° (Fig. 5.7).
3. The tape continues under the medial longitudinal arch to end on the superomedial aspect of the first ray. This will plantarflex the first ray when weight-bearing and reinforces the tape tension (Fig. 5.8).
4. Repeat with another support strip, overlapping the previous one by two-thirds (Fig. 5.9).
5. Finish with an anchor over the distal half of the first ray.

CHECK FUNCTION

When walking, the patient may feel a little unstable, as the ground contact surface area of the foot has been reduced with this taping procedure. The sensation quickly dissipates as the patient describes significant comfort, control and support with the technique.

CONTRAINDICATION

Do not apply for plantar fasciitis in the absence of rear foot pronation, or rigid feet with a normal or high-arch/cavus foot.

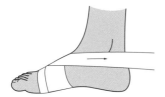

Figure 5.6

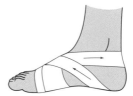

Figure 5.7

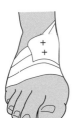

Figure 5.8

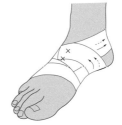

Figure 5.9

Tips

Apply this technique to the other side of the foot to promote calcaneal eversion, especially in the presence of a stiff subtalar joint.

Plantar fasciitis

H. Millson

INDICATION

Conditions such as plantar fasciitis/arch pain/medial tibial stress syndrome (MTSS) – chronic or acute.

FUNCTION

To support the arch and take pressure off the plantar fascia and thus allow healing.

MATERIALS

3.8-cm rigid or 3.8-cm stronger rigid tape (Leukotape P) and 5-cm elastic adhesive bandage (EAB).

POSITION

Sitting on the plinth with the foot relaxed over the edge of the bed.

APPLICATION

1. Apply the tape around the midfoot from lateral to medial, starting on the dorsum below the base of the fifth metatarsal and finishing on the dorsum below the base of the first metatarsal. **Note: Do not pull the strap. Place it around the foot.**
2. Leave a gap between the two edges of the tape on the dorsum of the foot, i.e. do not encircle the entire foot (Fig. 5.10a and b).
3. Repeat four to five times (dependent on the size of the foot), overlapping each strap by half (Fig. 5.11). **Note: It is critical that the last strap does not end at the origin of the plantar fascia on the calcaneum. This will aggravate the plantar fascia.**
4. The last strap may end on/around the medial malleolus to keep the underfoot area in a straight line throughout and thus prevent any wrinkles underfoot (Fig. 5.12).
5. Note that the taping does not extend far into the heel. It is just posterior to the plantar fascia origin on the calcaneus.
6. Apply two lock strips to tie down the loose ends on the dorsum of the foot, leaving a gap in the centre (Fig. 5.13).

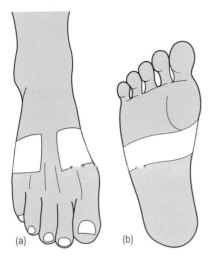

(a)   (b)

Figure 5.10

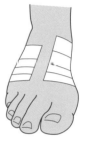

Figure 5.11

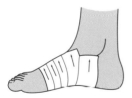

Figure 5.12

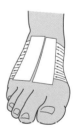

Figure 5.13

7. The strapping can be finished off with one or two lightly applied 5-cm EAB around the existing strapping, finishing on the dorsum of the foot. A small strip of rigid tape can be used to hold the EAB down (Fig. 5.14).

CHECK FUNCTION

Allow the patient to walk/run with taping and assess. Sometimes the taping needs to be reinforced during a match, e.g. rugby.

CAUTION

• The tape must **NOT** be pulled around the foot (lateral to medial) so that there is any change in the biomechanics of the foot.
• The tape must not terminate at the origin of the plantar fascia at the calcaneum.

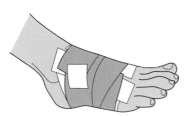

Figure 5.14

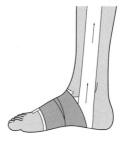

Figure 5.15

Note

If the patient has MTSS as a result of an overpronated foot, this tape can be used exactly as described. However, the last two straps may be brought up even further to travel along and finish at the junction of the medial shin and the muscle bulk, as high up as the MTSS pain (Fig. 5.15).

Tips

A stronger, more rigid tape (Leocotape P) can be used for the larger patient or the more demanding sport/conditions.
This tape is excellent as a temporary measure for assessing whether a patient needs medial arch supports (orthotics) as a permanent fixture.

Low dye taping

R. Macdonald

INDICATION

Overuse syndromes such as plantar fasciitis, medial arch strain, shin splints associated with overpronation.

FUNCTION

Limit abnormal pronation, reduce strain on the plantar fascia.

MATERIALS

Adhesive spray, 2.5-cm or 3.8-cm tape (width appropriate for foot size).

POSITION

The leg extended over end of couch, the foot relaxed.

APPLICATION

1. Spray the foot area to be taped.
2. Place tape on the lateral aspect of the fifth metatarsal head, draw the tape firmly along the lateral border of the foot and around the heel (Fig. 5.16).
3. Depress the first metatarsal head with the index finger, supporting the second to fifth metatarsal heads with the thumb (Fig. 5.17).
4. Draw the tape along the medial border and attach to the first metatarsal head (Fig. 5.18).
5. Repeat these strips once or twice more, overlapping the preceding strip by one-third.
6. Tie these strips down with two to three support tapes under the arch, from lateral to medial (Fig. 5.19).
7. Stand the athlete and close off the top of the foot with two to three bridging tapes while weight-bearing (Fig. 5.20).

CHECK FUNCTION

Does the foot feel more comfortable on weight-bearing?

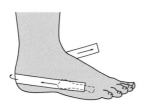
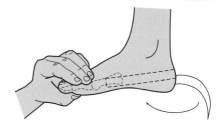

Figure 5.16

Figure 5.17

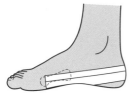
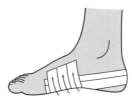

Figure 5.18

Figure 5.19

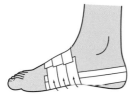

Figure 5.20

Tips

Do not extend the tapes across the joint line as this will 'splay' the first and fifth toes.
A heel wedge may be placed under the heel to aid supination.

Plantar fasciitis support

R. Macdonald

INDICATION

Longitudinal arch strain, overpronation (plantar fasciitis).

FUNCTION

To support the arch and relieve strain on the plantar fascia.

MATERIALS

5-cm stretch tape, 3.75-cm tape.

POSITION

Lying prone with the foot in neutral position over the end of the couch.

APPLICATION

Support

1. Using 5-cm stretch tape, start on the medial side of the foot, proximal to the head of the first metatarsal. Draw the tape along the medial border, around the heel and across the sole of the foot. Finish at the starting point (Fig. 5.21).
2. Repeat the procedure. Start proximal to the head of the fifth metatarsal. Draw the tape along the lateral border of the foot, around the heel and back to the starting point (applying tension as the tape passes over the plantar fascia attachment to the calcaneus; Fig. 5.22).

Cover strips

3. Fill in the sole of the foot with strips of stretch tape. Start at the metatarsal heads on the lateral side. Draw the tape towards the medial side. Lift the arch up before attaching medially (Fig. 5.23).

Lock strips

4. Secure edges by applying a strip of 3.75-cm tape from the fifth metatarsal head around the heel. Finish at the first metatarsal head (Fig. 5.24).
5. Stand the patient up. Apply one lock strip over the dorsum of the foot to secure the tape ends (Fig. 5.25).

CHECK FUNCTION

Check that the great toe and little toe are not splayed. If they are, release the edges.

CONTRAINDICATION

Rigid foot, pes planus.

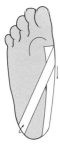

Figure 5.21

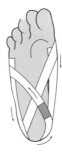

Figure 5.22

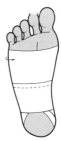

Figure 5.23

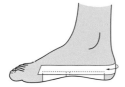

Figure 5.24

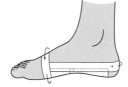

Figure 5.25

> **Tips**
>
> Apply slight stretch to the tape on application. A heel pad (Cyriax) is also beneficial.
>
> For a sweaty foot, apply the last lock strips around the whole foot, making sure that the forefoot is splayed (weight-bearing) before closing the ends on the dorsum of the foot.

Medial arch support

R. Macdonald

INDICATION

Medial longitudinal arch pain or overpronation.

FUNCTION

To lift and support the medial arch and relieve stress on the supporting ligaments.

MATERIALS

Felt or dense foam for arch pad, 7.5-cm or 10-cm stretch tape, 2.5-cm tape.

POSITION

Lying prone with the foot over the end of the couch.

APPLICATION

1. Measure the distance from the first metatarsal head to the anterior aspect of the calcaneus (Fig. 5.26). Cut an arch pad to fit this size and of appropriate thickness to raise the arch. Bevel the side of the pad which lies along the midline of the plantar surface of the foot. Sit the patient up on the couch.

Anchor

2. Using 7.5-cm or 10-cm stretch tape, depending on the size of the foot, cut a strip to wrap around the midfoot. Apply with minimal tension, with the adhesive side facing out. Ensure the closing seam is under the arch (this avoids seams under laces). Place the pad in position with the straight edge along the midline of the foot (Fig. 5.27).

Support strip

3. Cover with another strip of stretch tape, this time with the adhesive side innermost (Fig. 5.28).

Lock strip

4. Secure the seam with tape. Remove the entire support – turn inside out and close off the inside seam (Fig. 5.29).

CHECK FUNCTION

Allow the patient to move the support into a position of maximum support.

CONTRAINDICATION

Not to be worn in conjunction with a shoe containing a built-up medial arch support.

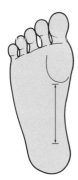

Figure 5.26

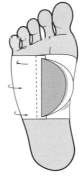

Figure 5.27

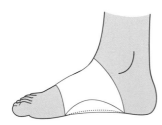

Figure 5.28

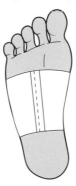

Figure 5.29

Tips

A removable support may be placed in the most comfortable position by the patient. Talcum powder will eliminate tackiness on an uncovered adhesive mass.

Cuboid subluxation in dancers

R. Macdonald

INDICATION

Minor subluxation of the cuboid associated with inversion ankle sprain in dancers, hypermobility of the calcaneocuboid joint on the plantar surface.

FUNCTION

To maintain the cuboid in a stable position and stabilize the midfoot.

MATERIALS

5-cm, 7.5-cm stretch tape, 3.8-cm rigid tape, felt adhesive pad.

POSITION

Seated with the foot over the edge of the couch.

APPLICATION

1. Stick the pad directly under the cuboid on the plantar surface of the foot with the outer edge bevelled.
2. Using 5-cm stretch tape, start on the medial side of the foot and draw the tape back and around the heel.
3. Angle the tape down the lateral side, under the arch, pull up and encircle the foot to finish under the arch (Fig. 5.30).
4. Repeat the procedure starting on the lateral side of the foot, passing around the heel, under the arch from the medial side, and encircling the foot to finish under the arch (Fig. 5.31).
5. Hold in place with one or two strips of 7.5-cm stretch tape around the midfoot.
6. Tie down the edge with a strip of 3.8-cm rigid tape.

CHECK FUNCTION

Stand the patient up to see if the technique is comfortable.

CONTRAINDICATION

Refrain from activity for a few days to avoid a recurrent subluxation.

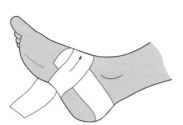

Figure 5.30

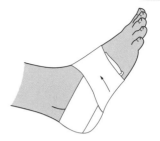

Figure 5.31

Heel pain

W.A. Hing and D.A. Reid

INDICATION

Heel pain, chronic plantar fasciitis, subtalar joint dysfunction. When a mobilization with movement (MWM) of the calcaneum has restored pain-free function (this may be internal or external rotation, depending on which direction relieves the pain).

FUNCTION

Alters the position of the calcaneum in relation to the talus, thus correcting a positional fault.

MATERIALS

Spray adhesive or hypoallergenic undertape (Fixomull or Mefix), 3.8-cm strapping tape.

POSITION

With the patient side-lying on the plinth with the ankle relaxed in neutral position. If taping to maintain internal rotation of the calcaneum, the patient lies with the affected ankle underneath, with the medial aspect of the ankle superior.

APPLICATION

Calcaneum taped into internal rotation.
1. The initial strip of tape is placed obliquely, around the back of the heel, while internal rotation of the calcaneum is maintained (Fig. 5.32).
2. Run the tape obliquely and medially over the calcaneum.
3. A second tape is placed over the first for effectiveness.

CHECK FUNCTION

When the patient initially stands, initial difficulty in walking may be experienced due to the repositioning of the calcaneum. Assess the original painful movements (i.e. weight-bearing and gait). Movements should now have pain-free full range of motion and function.

CONTRAINDICATION

If taping causes changes or an increase in pain. In particular, with this taping, tape should be left on overnight, as it is often in the morning that the patient feels most pain.

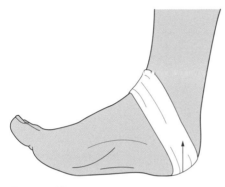

Figure 5.32

Tips

Easy to apply with the patient in the correct position; patients may be taught how to self-treat.

Heel contusion

R. Macdonald

INDICATION

Thinning of the fat pad due to trauma, overuse or lack of shock-absorbing material in the shoe.

FUNCTION

To compress the thinning fat pad from the edges toward the centre of the heel.

MATERIALS

Sponge rubber heel pad, adhesive spray, 2.5-cm tape.

POSITION

Prone with the feet over the edge of the couch.

APPLICATION

1. Spray the area and apply the pad to the base of the heel (may be applied before or after the tape job; Fig. 5.33).
2. Apply two anchors of tape interlocking around the heel and under the foot in a basketweave fashion (Fig. 5.34).
3. Repeat these strips overlapping the preceding ones by half, anchoring the pad in place.
4. The last strips should conform to the shape of the heel (Fig. 5.35).
5. Reapply the anchors (Fig. 5.36).

CHECK FUNCTION

Can the patient dorsiflex and plantarflex comfortably. Does the tape job take pressure off the bruise?

CONTRAINDICATION

Open wound on the heel base.

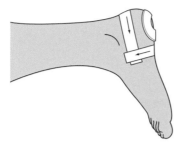

Figure 5.33

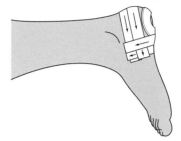

Figure 5.34

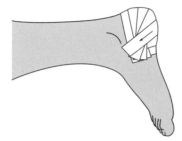

Figure 5.35

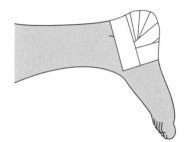

Figure 5.36

Tips

If available, a plastic heel cup may be used to compress the fat pad further, thus causing an air cushion under the heel.
A further strip of tape may be applied around the point of the heel to prevent the tape rolling when putting on a sock or shoe. Reapply anchors.

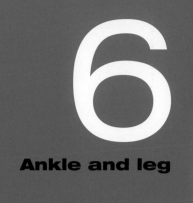

6

Ankle and leg

CHAPTER CONTENTS

Acute ankle sprain – field wrap

R. Macdonald

INDICATION

Immediate cohesive wrap for acute ankle sprain.

FUNCTION

To compress the injured soft tissue, help stop bleeding and contain swelling.

MATERIALS

7.5-cm cohesive elastic bandage.

POSITION

Seated with the leg supported and the foot in neutral position.

APPLICATION

For an inversion sprain:
1. Starting on the dorsum of the foot, encircle the foot once by taking the wrap down the medial side, under the arch and up the lateral side. Before encircling the foot a second time, fold down a corner of the first turn so that it will be locked in place on the second turn (Fig. 6.1).
2. Continue the wrap from the dorsum around the back of the heel, over the dorsum again, down the medial side under the heel, as far back on the heel as possible (Fig. 6.2).
3. As you come up on the lateral side, rip the bandage down the centre to just under the tip of the lateral malleolus and wrap one tail around the front of the ankle and the other around the back (Fig. 6.3).
4. The cohesive bandage will stick to itself; there is no need for pins or clasps.

CHECK FUNCTION

If the patient is unable to weight bear, a fracture must not be ruled out.

CONTRAINDICATION

Suspected fracture or total disruption.

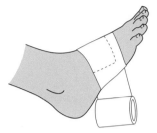

Figure 6.1

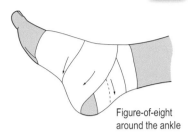

Figure-of-eight
around the ankle

Figure 6.2

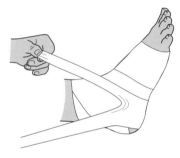

Figure 6.3

Tips

This wrap may be applied quickly and effectively on the field, as there
is no need for scissors or clamps to close off the technique. It can also
be applied over a shoe if removal of the shoe may cause further damage
to the injured structures.

Acute ankle sprain – open basketweave

R. Macdonald

INDICATION

Acute ankle sprain – inversion/eversion.

FUNCTION

Provide a more rigid support to a recently sprained ankle.

MATERIALS

Adhesive spray, underwrap, foam padding, 3.75-cm tape.

POSITION

Sitting with the foot and ankle over the edge of the plinth in neutral position.

APPLICATION

1. Spray area – apply a single layer of underwrap, spray foam pads, allow to get tacky, then apply around the medial and lateral malleoli.
2. Apply a half anchor to the leg about 10 cm above the malleoli and another around the foot posterior to the metatarsal heads. Do not close the anchors – leave a gap to allow swelling to subside. Apply a vertical strip from the medial side of the leg anchor, passing under the heel and up to attach to the lateral side. Apply a horizontal strip running from the lateral side of the foot anchor, around the heel and attach to the medial side (Fig. 6.4).
3. Apply two or three more strips in this fashion until the ankle joint is supported (Fig. 6.5).
4. Fill in with support strips from proximal to distal, again leaving a gap.
5. Cover the edges with two vertical strips running from top to bottom to finish (Fig. 6.6).

CHECK FUNCTION

Check that the foot is comfortable and supported on weight-bearing.

CONTRAINDICATION

Not able to weight bear.

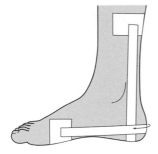

Figure 6.4

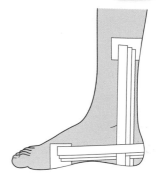

Figure 6.5

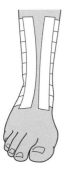

Figure 6.6

Tips

May be applied over a compression bandage for extra support.

Acute ankle sprain

W.A. Hing and D.A. Reid

INDICATION

Acutely swollen ankle following inversion sprain.

FUNCTION

To provide a degree of support to enhance early weight-bearing and to reduce the swelling, apply compression and give some lateral support.

MATERIALS

3.8-cm tape, shaver, Mylanta, Fixomull, orthopaedic felt, compressive bandage (Coban).

POSITION

Patient sitting with the ankle as close to neutral position as possible.

APPLICATION

1. Cut a felt horseshoe to fit around the lateral aspect of the ankle (Fig. 6.7).
2. Take a piece of 3.8-cm sports tape. Apply an anchor around the lower third of the leg (Fig. 6.8). This should not be tight or it will impede the flow of blood back up the leg.
3. Take another piece of sports tape. Attach to the anchor medially, working from medial to lateral to form a U-shaped stirrup. This keeps the tension toward the lateral side and prevents the ankle from turning in. In the acute stage, approximately two pieces of tape should be enough. Apply a final anchor over the top portion of the tape to hold the lateral tapes firm.
4. Finally, apply a Coban (cohesive bandage) over the taped ankle (Fig. 6.9). Start at the midfoot and apply a little more tension on the foot section, and reduce the tension as you work up the leg. This will ensure that the blood supply is enhanced in a distal to proximal direction.

CONTRAINDICATION

Excessive swelling and a patient unable to weight bear following injury – assess for risk of potential fracture.

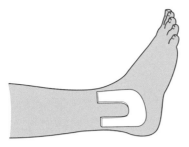

Figure 6.7

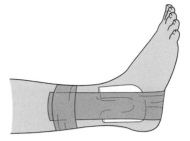

Figure 6.8

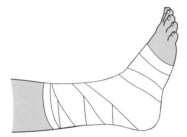

Figure 6.9

Tips

To enhance this, the use of a felt horseshoe increases the compression and supports the lateral ligament.

Also compresses the swelling around the lateral malleolus.

Inferior tibiofibular joint

W.A. Hing and D.A. Reid

INDICATION

Inversion trauma of the ankle resulting in a positional fault of the inferior tibiofibular joint. When a mobilization with movement (MWM) has restored pain-free function.

FUNCTION

Corrects the positional fault of the fibula by repositioning it back on the tibia. The injury occurs due to the fibula being forced forward during excessive inversion action.

MATERIALS

Spray adhesive or hypoallergenic undertape (Fixomull or Mefix), 3.8-cm strapping tape.

POSITION

Patient lying supine on the plinth with the ankle in neutral position.

APPLICATION

1. The aim of taping is to glide the fibula dorsocranially.
2. Apply and maintain MWM to the distal fibula.
3. The tape starts anterolaterally over the distal end of the fibula and lies obliquely (Fig. 6.10).
4. Direct the tape in a posterosuperior direction, making sure to lay the tape over the Achilles, to end anteromedially on the tibia (Fig. 6.11).

CHECK FUNCTION

Taping should not restrict ankle movements. Assess original painful movements (ankle inversion, gait). Movements should now be pain-free with full range of motion and function.

CONTRAINDICATION

In acute stages, ensure that taping does not prevent a reduction in swelling by being too tight or encompassing the leg. Also rule out the possibility of an avulsion fracture of the fibula.

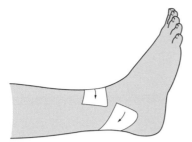

Figure 6.10

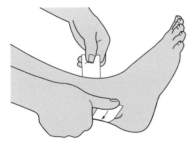

Figure 6.11

Tips

Never tape the foot in eversion, as this will inhibit normal ankle movement and thus slow down the healing process.
If taping causes changes or an increase in pain, it should not be left on for more than 48 h, and should be removed at any hint of skin irritation.

Ankle dorsiflexion and rear foot motion control

G. Lapenskie

INDICATION

Achilles tendon problems, subtalar motion problems:

• Achilles tendinitis.
• Subtalar instabilities following inversion ankle sprains.

FUNCTION

To control the amount of dorsiflexion of the ankle. To maintain the position of the rear foot during weight-bearing.

MATERIALS

Adhesive spray, 3.8-cm tape, 7.5-cm stretch tape.

POSITION

Put the athlete prone, lying with the foot extending beyond the bed. Place the rear foot in the desired position.

APPLICATION

1. Start a piece of 3.8-cm tape on the distal third, medial aspect of the leg. Bring the tape down and laterally over the lateral aspect of the heel, under the arch, to the dorsum of the foot (Fig. 6.12).
2. Start a second piece of 3.8-cm tape on the lateral aspect of the leg at the distal third of the leg. Bring the tape medially over the medial aspect of the heel, under the arch, to the dorsum of the foot (Fig. 6.13).
3. Repeat the sequence three times in each direction, slightly overlapping towards the midline of the leg (Fig. 6.14).

Anchor strips

4. Anchor the proximal and distal ends of the tape with the 7.5-cm stretch tape (Fig. 6.15).

CHECK FUNCTION

Is the tape irritating the Achilles tendon during gait?

CONTRAINDICATION

Acute peritendinitis.

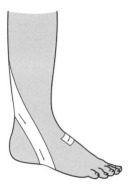

Figure 6.12

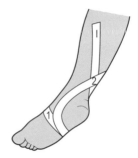

Figure 6.13

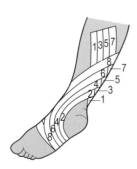

Figure 6.14

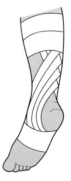

Figure 6.15

Tips

Place a heel cushion under the heel.

Achilles tendinopathy

W.A. Hing and D.A. Reid

INDICATION

Pain on the medial or lateral aspect of the tendon. When a MWM has restored pain-free function.

FUNCTION

Utilized when the patient has pronated or supinated feet. In the case of pronated feet (when viewed from behind), the Achilles tendon may appear convex medially and thus more vulnerable to strain.

Taping reduces the loading on the medial aspect of the tendon by making the tendon concave medially, alters the way the foot weight bears and changes the tracking of the tendon/muscle.

MATERIALS

Spray adhesive or hypoallergenic undertape (Fixomull or Mefix), 3.8-cm strapping tape, shaver.

POSITION

Patient lying prone with the foot relaxed over the edge of the plinth.

APPLICATION

Taping for medial Achilles tendon pain:
1. Apply tape to the medial aspect of the tendon, running posteriorly.
2. Place a finger on the medial aspect of the tendon over the tape and apply lateral pressure to concave the tendon medially, thus correcting the convexity.
3. Direct the tape posteriorly, 'laying on' over the tendon and continuing around the lateral aspect of the ankle to finish anteriorly (Fig. 6.16).
4. Once the initial piece of tape has been applied, lay a second piece directly over the first.

CHECK FUNCTION

The tendon should appear in neutral, or concave to the side of the painful tendon once taped. Assess original painful movements (i.e. walking, toe raise). Movements should now have pain-free full range of motion and function.

CONTRAINDICATION

If taping causes changes or an increase in pain, tape should not be left on for more than 48 h, and should be removed at any hint of skin irritation.

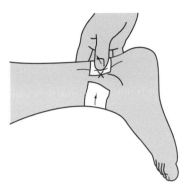

Figure 6.16

Tips

Use Mylanta (this is a stomach antacid which neutralizes the acidity of the tape – use extra strength) on the skin to avoid an adverse skin reaction to the tape. Before applying the tape, brush off the surface powder that appears when the Mylanta dries.

This procedure is easy to apply with the patient in the correct position, so a family member could be taught to do the taping. This would allow the tape to be removed at night and reapplied in the morning, preventing the risk of an adverse skin reaction.

Achilles tendinopathy

H. Millson

INDICATION

Acute or chronic pain/tenderness on all or any part of the Achilles tendon. To be used as an adjunct to treatment of the Achilles tendon, in particular specific soft tissue massage (SSTM). To be used with bilateral heel raises.

FUNCTION

To reduce the load on the Achilles tendon when walking, exercising or playing any sport.

MATERIALS

Friars Balsam adhesive protective lotion, rigid tape: 3.8 cm or extra strong rigid tape (Leukotape P), stretch tape: can use hypoallergenic undertape (Fixomull) if allergic or hypersensitive.

POSITION

Patient lying prone with the foot relaxed but in slight plantarflexion (this position of plantarflexion can be altered according to the patient's functional demands/individual response; however, it must not be in too much plantarflexion). A small pillow under the lower leg.

APPLICATION

1. Apply an anchor using 7.5-cm elastic adhesive bandage (EAB) to the lower leg, two-thirds of the way up the calf on the gastrocnemius muscle bulk.
2. Apply a second anchor using 5-cm EAB around the midfoot, making sure that the tape ends on the dorsum of the foot. Use a small strip of rigid tape to hold the ends of the EAB down.
3. Start the Achilles tendon strap using 5-cm EAB tape, the length being from anchor to anchor:
   - Split the tape for about 4 cm at both ends, giving you four tails (Fig. 6.17).
   - Apply the tails to the anchors, i.e. two to the calf anchor medial and lateral (Fig. 6.18a) and two to the plantar aspect of the foot anchor (Fig. 6.18b). The strapping does not touch the skin along the length of the Achilles.
   - Fold the strap along its length from the V to the V to make a firm vertical line (Fig. 6.19a).

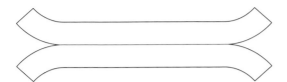

Figure 6.17

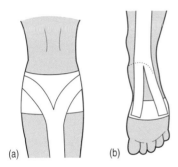

(a) (b)

Figure 6.18

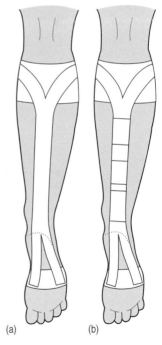

(a) (b)

Figure 6.19

- Apply small strips of rigid tape horizontally around the strapping line to 'close' and strengthen the strap (Fig. 6.19b).
4. A second tape may be applied over the first for further strength. One could use rigid tape over the EAB down the length of the calf in order to strengthen it further. This is dependent upon the size of the patient/the patient's sporting demands/the type of playing surface.
5. Apply EAB around the two anchors to hold them in place. This must not constrict the calf/foot (Fig. 6.20).
6. The vertical 'Achilles tendon strap' is neat and off the skin. It should lie in a direct line with the Achilles tendon (Fig. 6.21). It does not rub against the heel at all. However, if this is the case, a piece of gauze may be placed around the heel.

CHECK FUNCTION

This step is vital! Let the patient walk/run/sport specific movement with the taping and he/she will be able to assess the comfort immediately. The tape can easily be adjusted (even by the patient) by removing the top EAB cover and pulling the V-shape tape higher/further onto the anchor on each side. This will immediately shorten the vertical tape and tighten the strap.

CAUTION

Take care that the foot is not in too much plantarflexion, that the vertical strap is not too short and that the anchor and closing straps are not too tight around the calf. There should be no gaps or wrinkles.

CONTRAINDICATION

Any skin allergies. Any pain after taping.

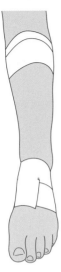

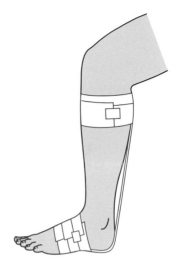

Figure 6.20

Figure 6.21

Tips

An even stronger rigid tape can be used for the larger patient or the more demanding sport/conditions. The patient can be taught to adjust the tape (as stated above) before or during the activity of daily living/ sporting activity.

Achilles tendon support – two methods

O. Rouillon

INDICATION

1. Simple method – using stretch tape, non-weight-bearing, preventive.
2. To stabilize the rear foot, preventive.
3. Rigid tape method – for sport.
   Prophylactically, it is better to use type 1 or 2.

Method 1 – simple method

MATERIALS

Gauze squares, lubricant, adhesive spray, prowrap, scissors (blunt-ended), 8-cm and 6-cm stretch tape.

POSITION

Sitting with the leg over the end of the couch.

APPLICATION

Lubricated gauze square over the Achilles tendon. Adhesive spray on the leg. Prowrap from the foot to the top of the calf.
1. Using 6-cm stretch tape, apply an anchor around the foot, proximal to the metatarsal heads, and another around the proximal end of the calf.

Second position

Prone lying:
2. Using 6-cm stretch tape, attach it to the distal anchor on the plantar surface. Pass over the calcaneum and Achilles tendon and attach to the posterior aspect of the proximal anchor, with tension (Fig. 6.22).
3. Attach two more strips to the plantar surface, bisecting strip 1. Pass upwards to the proximal anchor with the inner edge travelling along the centre of strip 1, one each on the medial and lateral aspects (Fig. 6.23).
4. Using 8-cm stretch tape, attach it centrally on the distal anchor. Proceed as before up the posterior aspect of the calf. Before attaching, cut two tails at the proximal end, 20 cm long. Separate at the musculotendinous junction of the triceps surae; attach to the proximal anchor medially and laterally to the previous strips (Fig. 6.24).
Finish by repeating the original anchors (lock strips) proximal and distal.

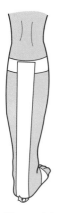

Figure 6.22

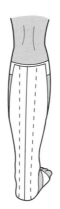

Figure 6.23

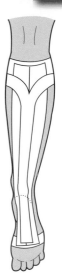

Figure 6.24

Method 2 – for rear foot stabilization

MATERIALS

Two gauze squares for the Achilles tendon and the anterior foot tendons, spray, prowrap and lubricant.

POSITION

Proceed as for method 1.

APPLICATION

Using 6-cm stretch tape, apply two anchors, one around the midfoot, the second around the proximal calf.

Anchors

1. Cut three strips of 6-cm tape, measuring from the proximal to the distal anchor. Attach to the proximal anchor. Cut two tails on the distal end, 10 cm long. Split the tails to just above the Achilles tendon.
2. Apply the medial tail over the medial malleoli under the calcaneum, up the lateral side of the foot to finish on the dorsum. Repeat with the other tail, passing over the lateral aspect.
3. Apply the second and third strips in the same manner, superimposed on strip 1, moving anteriorly (Fig. 6.25).

Finish

Apply 6-cm cohesive wrap.

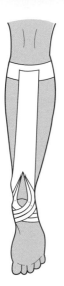

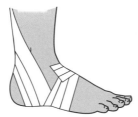

Figure 6.25

Tips

Cut three strips before you start.

Preventive taping for injuries to the lateral aspect of the ankle joint

D. Reese

INDICATION

- Prevention of injuries caused by foot inversion.
- Strain to the peroneus tendons.
- Slight or healing sprain to the anterior talofibular ligament and/or calcaneofibular ligament.

FUNCTION

To give support to the lateral aspect of the ankle by a combination of mechanical support supplied by the tape and its interface with the anchors, and proprioceptive response triggered by the pull of the skin when supinating the foot during activity.

MATERIALS

3.75-cm or 5-cm tape, depending on the size of the ankle. Underwrap and one or two gauze squares with lubricant.

POSITION

Patient sitting with the foot over the end of the bench or the lower leg supported by a taping support under the lower leg.

APPLICATION

The patient should be clean, dry and shaved in the area to be taped. Start by having the patient actively holding the foot neutrally at the anatomical 0 position for the foot (or 90°). For patients who sweat profusely or who will be active in a wet environment, it is recommended to use adhesive spray. Apply the underwrap in a figure-of-eight around the ankle joint, covering the lower aspect of the Achilles tendon and the dorsal aspect of the joint, or place two heel-and-lace pads or gauze squares with lubricant (one placed on the Achilles tendon, the other at the dorsal junction between the malleoli and the talus).

Anchors

Anchors 1, 2 and 3 should be placed starting approximately 5 cm distal to the belly of the gastrocnemius. Apply the tape so that it conforms to the natural angle of the lower leg. Overlap distally approximately one-quarter of the width of the first anchor. The bottom part of the last anchor should lie just proximal to the malleoli. Check to see that the anchors do not constrict the range of motion (Fig. 6.26).

Support

1. The first support should start just proximal to the lateral malleolus. It should be angled downward towards the posterior aspect of the calcaneus and then pulled tautly upward, covering the back half of the lateral malleolus and continuing upward to the level of the first anchor (Fig. 6.27).
2. The second support starts proximal to the first support. The angle downward should be directed so that, as it passes anteriorly to the medial malleolus, it should lie directly on top of the first support, continuing on the calcaneus, to be pulled tautly upward covering the anterior half of the malleolus, and creating a V-formation together with the first support (Fig. 6.28).
3. The third support is placed in the centre of the first two. Pull tautly upward, covering the malleolus (Fig. 6.29).

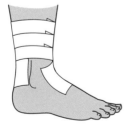
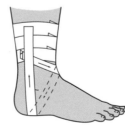
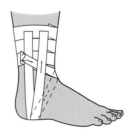

Figure 6.26   **Figure 6.27**   **Figure 6.28**

Anchor lock

Apply three more anchors over the originals (Fig. 6.30).

Anchor support

The arch support should start proximal to the medial malleolus. It passes downward over the lateral aspect of the foot and then is pulled tautly upward, finishing at the apex of the medial arch (Fig. 6.31).

Heel lock

The lateral heel lock starts proximal to the lateral malleolus. It should be angled downward towards the posterior aspect of the calcaneum and then pulled tautly upward, covering the calcaneum laterally. It continues over the medial malleolus, angled upward, and finishes parallel to the start (Fig. 6.32).

CHECK FUNCTION

Once the supports have been applied, hold them manually in place and ask the patient if he or she is receiving the desired support. If not, adjust the supports before applying the anchor locks.

CONTRAINDICATION

Application should be avoided when the patient has a swollen joint.

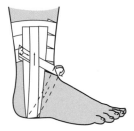

Figure 6.29

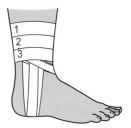

Figure 6.30

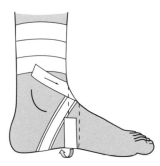

Figure 6.31

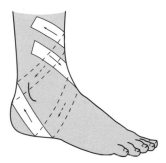

Figure 6.32

Tips

Best applied directly to the skin. When applying the supports, be careful to keep proximal to the base of the fifth metatarsal.

Closed basketweave taping for the ankle

R. Macdonald

INDICATION

Ankle inversion sprain.

FUNCTION

To support the lateral ligaments without limiting motion unnecessarily.

MATERIALS

Gauze squares or heel-and-lace pads, petroleum jelly, adhesive spray, underwrap, 3.75-cm tape.

POSITION

Patient sitting on the couch/bench with the foot and ankle over the edge, the foot in dorsiflexion and everted.

APPLICATION

Spray the area. Apply lubricated gauze squares over pressure areas (extensor tendons and Achilles tendon). Apply a single layer of underwrap (Fig. 6.33).

Anchors

Apply anchors to the leg about 10 cm above the malleoli, conforming to the shape of the leg, and to the midfoot. These anchors should overlap the underwrap by 2 cm and adhere directly to the skin (Fig. 6.34).

Support

Apply first the vertical stirrup, starting on the medial side of the anchor. Continue down posterior to the medial malleolus, under the heel and up the lateral side (with tension). Attach to the anchor. (Do not mould to leg.)

Horizontal strips

Apply a horizontal (Gibney) strip. Start on the lateral side of the anchor, continue around the heel and attach to the medial side of the foot anchor (Fig. 6.35). Continue to apply vertical and horizontal strips alternately until

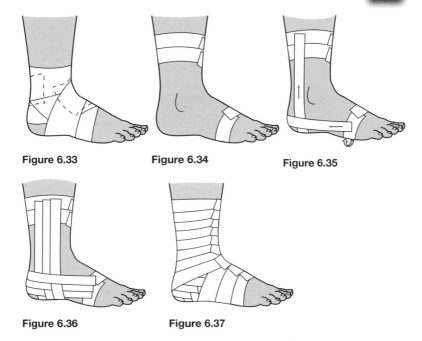

Figure 6.33

Figure 6.34

Figure 6.35

Figure 6.36

Figure 6.37

the ankle is covered. Ensure each strip overlaps the preceding one by one-third (Fig. 6.36).

Lock strips

Fill in with locking strips between the anchors (Fig. 6.37).

CHECK FUNCTION

Is it supportive, but not too tight?

CONTRAINDICATION

Swelling, inflammation, bleeding.

Tips
Mould with hands to warm and set.

Heel locks for closed basketweave

R. Macdonald

INDICATION

Ankle sprain.

FUNCTION

To provide extra support with double heel lock.

MATERIALS

3.8-cm tape.

APPLICATION

1. Start on the medial side of the leg. Angle the tape down over the lateral side, behind and under the heel, pulling up and out (Fig. 6.38).
2. Continue over the dorsum of the foot, back over the medial malleolus behind the heel (Fig. 6.39).
3. Continue down under the heel, pulling up to the medial side (Fig. 6.40).
4. Proceed across the front of the foot and finish high on the lateral side (Fig. 6.41).

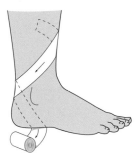

Figure 6.38

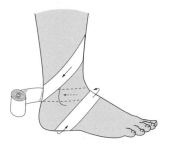

Figure 6.39

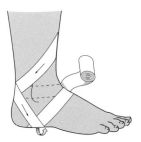

Figure 6.40

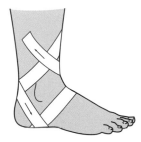

Figure 6.41

Tips

For the novice, two single heel locks are easier to apply. The first starts on the medial side, and the second on the lateral side.

Calcaneal motion control

G. Lapenskie

INDICATION

Subtalar motion problems following inversion ankle sprain:

• sinus tarsi pain
• referred Achilles tendon pain
• reflex peroneal weakness.

FUNCTION

To maintain the subtalar joint in the neutral position by eliminating excessive calcaneal excursion.

MATERIALS

Tape adherent, 2.5-cm stretch tape.

POSITION

The athlete is placed in a supine position.

APPLICATION

1. Position the calcaneus in the desired position.
2. To avoid excessive varus motion, cut a piece of stretch tape 30 cm in length, and place the mid portion of the tape on the medial aspect of the calcaneus. Bring the end of the tape close to the metatarsal heads under the arch of the foot, up the lateral aspect of the foot and over the dorsum of the foot, ending the tape by wrapping it around the lower leg. The piece nearest the calcaneus comes behind the calcaneus, anteriorly over the lateral malleolus, ending the tape by wrapping it around the lower leg (Figs 6.42 and 6.43).
3. Repeat step 2 (Fig. 6.44).

CHECK FUNCTION

Is the calcaneum stabilized when the patient is running (rear view)?

Figure 6.42

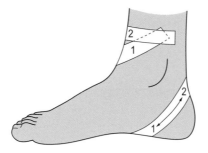

Figure 6.43

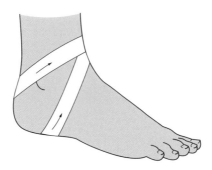

Figure 6.44

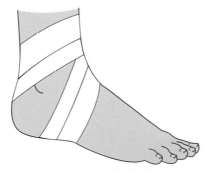

Tips

To avoid excessive valgus motion, start the tape on the lateral aspect of the calcaneus.

A heel pad is sometimes beneficial (Cyriax).

Superior tibiofibular joint

W.A. Hing and D.A. Reid

INDICATION

Posterolateral knee pain, commonly with weight-bearing and gait, especially walking down stairs or slopes. Patients with remnants of leg pain down the lateral border of the lower leg to the foot. Note the previously described conditions in which MWMs are pain-free and successful.

FUNCTION

Repositions the fibula head forward on the tibia. Also, possibly alters tension on the nerve responsible for pain (e.g. common peroneal nerve).

MATERIALS

Spray adhesive or hypoallergenic undertape (Fixomull or Mefix), 3.8-cm strapping tape, shaver.

POSITION

Patient standing with the affected knee flexed and the foot placed on a chair.

APPLICATION

1. Place tape over the superior head of the fibula.
2. Apply and maintain a MWM to the superior fibula head (Fig. 6.45).
3. In an anterior direction, wrap tape obliquely across the front of the tibia.
4. Tape will end on the medial side of the tibia (Fig. 6.46).

CHECK FUNCTION

Ensure there is full range of motion at the knee, and that the tape is not constricting the gastrocnemius muscles. Assess original painful movements (knee flexion, stepping down off a step). Movements should now have pain-free full range of motion and function.

CONTRAINDICATION

If taping causes changes or an increase in pain. Also tape should not be left on for more than 48 h, and should be removed at any hint of skin irritation.

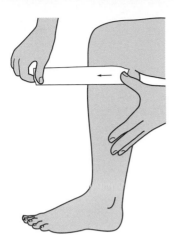

Figure 6.45

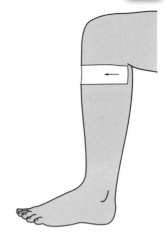

Figure 6.46

Tips

Easy to apply with the patient in the correct position, so the patient can be taught to do taping. This would allow the tape to be removed at night and reapplied in the morning, preventing the risk of an adverse skin reaction.

Medial tibial stress syndrome (MTSS) and antipronation taping

D. Morrissey

INDICATION

This technique is used for symptomatic relief during rehabilitation or sporting activity, alone or in combination with other antipronation measures such as low dye taping, antipronation insoles and muscle retraining.

FUNCTION

The aim is to reduce the symptoms and pronation.

MATERIALS

5-cm Mefix/Hypafix, 4-cm zinc oxide tape, elastic adhesive bandage.

POSITION

Standing or sitting with the foot on a slightly raised surface, the ankle in plantarflexion and the leg muscles relaxed.

APPLICATION

1. The Mefix is applied without tension to the anteromedial lower shin, then spirals laterally and upwardly around the posterior leg to finish on the anterior aspect just below the knee joint.
2. Two or three strips of zinc oxide are then applied over the Mefix, overlapping each other by one-third the width of the tape. These are used to pull the long flexors of the foot (flexor hallucis longus, flexor digitorum longus and tibialis posterior in particular) towards the medial tibial border. Applied with minimal tension, the tape effectively tightens on weight-bearing (Fig. 6.47).
3. Anchor and locking strips are then applied at the proximal and distal ends of the spiral using elastic adhesive bandage (Fig. 6.48).

CHECK FUNCTION

Check that gait is uninhibited.

CONTRAINDICATION

Allergic reaction, open skin wounds, excessive hair.

INSTRUCTIONS TO PATIENT

The tape may be left on for up to 12 h providing the skin is not red or itchy.

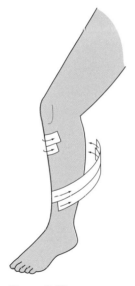

Figure 6.47

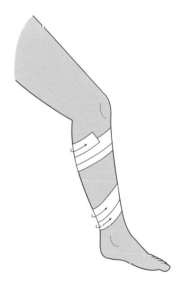

Figure 6.48

Tips

Shave the legs at least 24 h prior to taping.

7

Knee

chapter

CHAPTER CONTENTS

Patellar tendinosis

W.A. Hing and D.A. Reid

INDICATION

Patellar tendinosis, unloading the tendon or fat pad, also useful for managing the pain of Osgood–Schlatter's disease.

FUNCTION

Unload the tendon and reduce pain in the tendon or attachment.

MATERIALS

Spray adhesive or hypoallergenic undertape (Fixomull or Mefix), 3.8-cm strapping tape.

POSITION

Patient sitting with the knee in full extension.

APPLICATION

1. Place one anchor strap over the thigh just above the superior patellar pole.
2. Attach one strip of tape to the anchor on the medial side of the knee, and pull the tape obliquely downward to the lateral side with the top edge of the tape passing just under the inferior patellar pole.
3. Repeat this action from lateral to medial, to make a crossover effect, with the V of the cross in the midline just under the inferior patellar pole (Fig. 7.1).
4. Repeat this process until you have done two to three overlapping layers.
5. Do one final lock-off anchor over the top of the original anchor.

CHECK FUNCTION

When the patient stands and tries to bend the knee, there should be sufficient tension for the pressure to be felt over the tendon immediately under the knee cap.

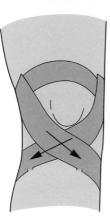

Figure 7.1

Tips

Use Mylanta (this is a stomach antacid which neutralizes the acidity of the tape; use extra strength) on the skin to avoid an adverse skin reaction to the tape. Before applying the tape, brush off the surface powder that appears when the Mylanta dries.

Unload the fat pad

J. McConnell

INDICATION

Inferior patellofemoral pain, hyperextended knees, irritated fat pad, post knee arthroscopy.

FUNCTION

Unloads an irritated fat pad.

MATERIALS

Hypoallergenic tape (Endurafix/Fixomull/Hypafix/Mefix) and 3.8-cm tape.

POSITION

Patient lying, leg relaxed.

APPLICATION

Apply the hypoallergenic tape to the area to be taped.
1. Commence tape on the superior part of the patella to tip the inferior pole out of the fat pad (Fig. 7.2).
2. The next tape starts at the tibial tuberosity and goes out wide to the medial knee joint. The soft tissue is lifted towards the patella (Fig. 7.3).
3. The final tape starts at the tibial tuberosity, going wide to the lateral joint line.

CHECK FUNCTION

Check painful activity, which should now be pain-free if the tape has been applied properly.

CONTRAINDICATION

Skin allergy – the skin must be protected prior to taping.

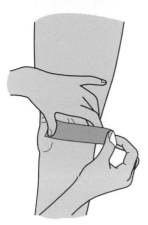

Figure 7.2

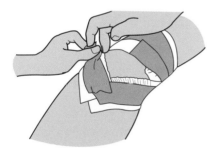

Figure 7.3

Tips

The skin should have an orange-peel look.
The patient should be discouraged from hyperextending the knee.

Knee support – Crystal Palace wrap

R. Macdonald

INDICATION

Retropatellar pain, jumper's knee and Osgood–Schlatter's disease.

FUNCTION

To relieve pressure of the patella on the femur. To relieve stress on the tibial tubercle.

MATERIALS

Gauze square, petroleum jelly, 5-cm or 7.5-cm stretch tape, 3.75-cm tape.

POSITION

Patient standing with the knee relaxed and slightly flexed.

APPLICATION

Cut a strip of stretch tape approximately 50 cm and place gauze in the centre.

Support strips

1. Lay tape on the back of the knee with the gauze square in the popliteal fossa. Mould the tape to the femoral condyles (Fig. 7.4).
2. Split the lateral strip into two tails. Stretch and twist the tails separately and attach to the medial condyle, passing over the patellar tendon in the soft spot between the inferior patellar pole and tibial tubercle (Fig. 7.5). Repeat with the second tail.
3. Stretch the medial strip across the twisted tails. Attach to the lateral condyle (Fig. 7.6).

Lock strips

4. Close off with tape strips (Fig. 7.7).

CHECK FUNCTION

Have the patient squat. Is it tight in the popliteal fossa?

CONTRAINDICATION

Not suitable for those with rotated patellar dysfunction.

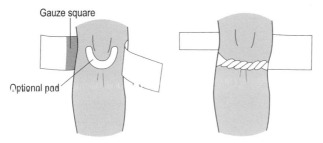

Gauze square

Optional pad

Figure 7.4

Figure 7.5

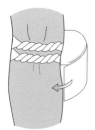

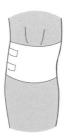

Figure 7.6

Figure 7.7

Tips

Best applied directly to the skin. Shave, wash and dry the skin. Apply skin prep on tough skin before taping.

Sprain of the lateral collateral ligament

O. Rouillon

FUNCTION

To provide basic lateral stabilization of the knee.

MATERIALS

Lubricant, gauze squares, adhesive spray, two rolls of 6-cm stretch tape, 15-cm stretch tape, 3.8-cm tape.

POSITION

The patient is standing with the knee in 15° flexion and the roll of tape under the heel. The leg is pushed laterally. Apply the gauze with lubricant to the popliteal fossa. Apply adhesive spray and prowrap.

APPLICATION

1. Using 6-cm stretch tape, apply two anchors to the lower third of the thigh and one anchor at the tibial tubercle (Fig. 7.8).
2. Using 6-cm stretch tape, apply a diagonal strip from the anteromedial aspect of the proximal anchor to the posteromedial aspect of the distal anchor.
3. The second symmetrical strip crosses the first at the centre of the medial joint line (Fig. 7.9).
4. Repeat this sequence with two more strips overlapping the previous strips by one-half anteriorly (Fig. 7.10).
5. Repeat the same sequence on the lateral knee joint.
6. Using six strips of 3.8-cm tape, apply a symmetrical montage, on top of the previous strips, with tension on the medial and lateral aspects of the knee joint (Fig. 7.11).
7. Lock the tape job in place with incomplete circles of tape (Fig. 7.12).
8. To protect the popliteal fossa, using a strip of 15-cm stretch tape, cut two tails on either end. Place the lubricated gauze square in the centre. Close the tails above and below the patellar poles (Fig. 7.13).
9. Finish with 6-cm stretch tape by reapplying the original anchors. Figure 7.14a shows the position of the leg for Figures 7.8 and 7.12, and Figure 7.14b shows the position of the leg for Figure 7.9.

CAUTION

Do not impinge the inferior patellar pole into the fat pad.

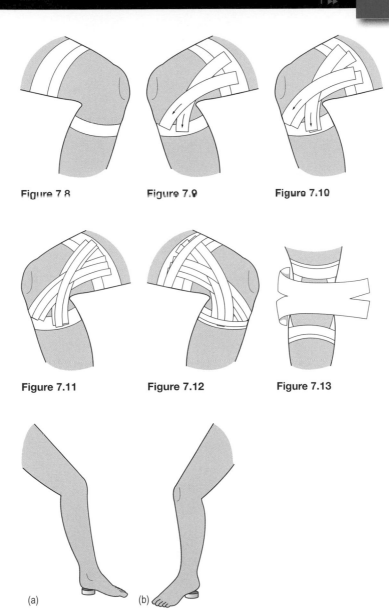

Figure 7.8

Figure 7.9

Figure 7.10

Figure 7.11

Figure 7.12

Figure 7.13

(a)

(b)

Figure 7.14

Anterior cruciate taping

K.E. Wright

INDICATION

Sprain to the anterior cruciate ligament of the knee.

FUNCTION

To provide support and stability to the knee's anterior cruciate ligament.

MATERIALS

3.8-cm adhesive tape, 7.5-cm elastic tape and gauze with lubricant.

POSITION

The knee and hip joints should be positioned in slight flexion.

APPLICATION

1. Apply gauze and lubricant to the posterior aspect of the knee joint. You should also apply an anchor strip of 7.5-cm elastic tape around the upper third of the thigh (Fig. 7.15). Note: in this pretaping procedure, do not compress the popliteal fossa.
2. Using 7.5-cm elastic tape, begin on the lower leg's lateral aspect, approximately 2.5 cm below the patella. Encircle the lower leg, move anteriorly then medially, continuing to the posterior aspect and returning to the lateral side. Angle the tape below the patella, cross the medial joint line and popliteal fossa, and spiral up to the anterior portion of the upper thigh's anchor (Fig. 7.16).
3. The next strip of 7.5-cm elastic tape will begin on the anterior aspect of the proximal anchor (Fig. 7.17) and cross the thigh's medial portion, covering the popliteal fossa, encircling the lower leg and crossing the popliteal fossa again. You will finish by spiralling up to the anterior aspect of the thigh's proximal anchor (Fig. 7.18).
4. Repeat step 3.
5. Secure this technique by applying 3.8-cm adhesive tape over the thigh's anchor (Fig. 7.19).

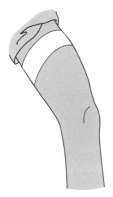

Figure 7.15

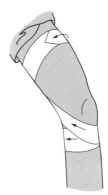

Figure 7.16

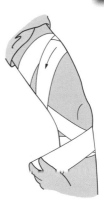

Figure 7.17

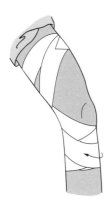

Figure 7.18

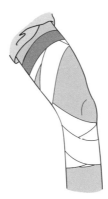

Figure 7.19

Continuous figure-of-eight wrap for the knee

K.E. Wright

INDICATION

Sprains to the knee joint.

FUNCTION

To provide support to the knee joint.

MATERIALS

10-cm elastic wrap, 3.8-cm adhesive tape.

POSITION

The knee joint placed in slight flexion.

APPLICATION

1. Begin the wrap on the lateral/posterior aspect of the lower leg. Encircle the lower leg, moving medially to laterally.
2. Angle the wrap below the patella and cross the medial joint line (Fig. 7.20). Cover the thigh's posterior and lateral aspect. Encircle the thigh, moving medially to laterally (Fig. 7.21). Angle the wrap downward, staying above the patella, and crossing the medial joint line (Fig. 7.22). Cross the popliteal space and encircle the lower leg (Fig. 7.23).
3. Proceed with the wrap, crossing the lateral joint line and angling above the patella (Fig. 7.24). Encircle the thigh and, on the posterior aspect, angle across the knee's lateral joint line, staying below the patella (Fig. 7.25). This configuration should resemble a diamond shape around the patella and cover from mid thigh to the gastrocnemius belly. Secure this wrap with 2.5-cm adhesive tape, applied at the wrap's loose end.

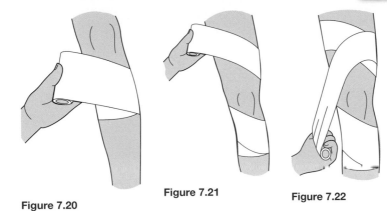

Figure 7.20

Figure 7.21

Figure 7.22

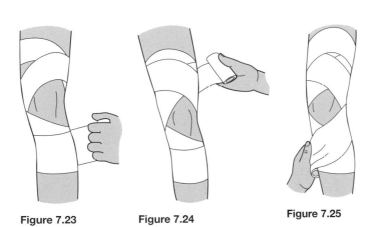

Figure 7.23

Figure 7.24

Figure 7.25

Vastus lateralis inhibitory technique

U. McCarthy Persson

INDICATION

Patellofemoral pain with an increased activity of the vastus lateralis (VL) muscle in relation to the vastus medialis obliquus. This technique can also be useful for other conditions in which a decrease in VL activity is desirable.

FUNCTION

The tape can decrease the muscle activity of the VL during weight-bearing activities and may restore balance of the quadriceps muscle function and decrease patellofemoral pain.

MATERIALS

3.8-cm rigid tape, 5-cm Fixomull or Hypafix hypoallergenic tape.

POSITION

Patient in side lying with a pillow between the knees, which are flexed to an angle of 30°.

APPLICATION

1. Two lengths of flexible hypoallergenic tape are applied without tension to the mid point of the thigh extending from the rectus femoris muscle laterally to the midline of the iliotibial band.
2. A total of three rigid zinc oxide tape strips are then applied, from proximal to distal, overlapping each other by one-third.
3. The three strips are applied with tension on top of the hypoallergenic tape from the anterior aspect laterally to the posterior aspect. The lateral thigh tissues are gathered with the other hand while applying a downward pressure with the thumb over the VL between the reference lines, causing a furrow in the skin (Fig 7.26).
4. The tension applied to the tape can be standardized to cause a 'skin roll' anterior and posterior to the thumb with the same height as the width of the therapist's thumb.

CHECK FUNCTION

Assess active movement, pain and muscle function. The tape should feel very tight when applied correctly.

CONTRAINDICATION

Ensure that the rigid tape does not extend beyond the hypoallergenic tape, thus avoiding possible skin irritation.

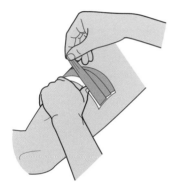

Figure 7.26

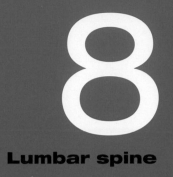

8 chapter ◀◀

Lumbar spine

CHAPTER CONTENTS

Lumbar spine taping

W.A. Hing and D.A. Reid

INDICATION

Lumbar dysfunction and pain. Avoidance of painful lumbar flexion or postures. Application following Mulligan lumbar sustained natural apophyseal glides (SNAGs) or McKenzie extensions.

FUNCTION

Maintains neutral to extended lumbar lordosis. Avoids pain-provoking positions and facilitates a more extended posture.

MATERIALS

Spray adhesive or hypoallergenic undertape (Fixomull or Mefix), 3.8-cm or 5-cm strapping tape.

POSITION

Patient lying prone or may be taped in sitting or standing. Patient must be able to achieve a relaxed and pain-free extended lumbar posture (lordosis) while the tape is being applied.

APPLICATION

1. Spine in neutral to slightly extended position with lumbar curvatures maintained.
2. Anchor strips are applied to the top and bottom of the area to be taped.
3. An X is formed across the lumbar region from the top anchor to the bottom anchor, with the centre of the X overlying the L2–3 region (Fig. 8.1). Repeat this X with two more strips overlapping the previous strips by half.
4. The top and bottom of the X are then reanchored.

CHECK FUNCTION

Assess original painful movements (i.e. flexion, reaching forward). Movements should now be pain-free and limited at end of range.

CONTRAINDICATION

Check skin reaction to the tape and tell the patient to remove it if an adverse skin reaction occurs. Tape should not be left on for more than 48 h.

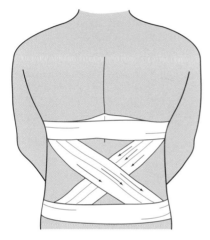

Figure 8.1

Tips

This procedure is easy to apply with the patient in the correct position, so a family member could be taught to do the taping. This would allow the tape to be removed at night and reapplied in the morning, preventing the risk of an adverse skin reaction.

Frontal plane pelvic stability

A. Hughes

INDICATION

Conditions aggravated by excessive lateral horizontal pelvic tilt, trochanteric bursitis, piriformis syndrome, sacroiliac joint (SIJ) instability, iliotibial band (ITB) friction syndrome or runner's knee, patellofemoral pain.

FUNCTION

To control excessive lateral horizontal pelvic tilt (Trendelenberg sign) and facilitate femoral external rotation to limit lateral and posterior displacement of the femoral greater trochanter in the stance phase.

MATERIALS

3.8-cm rigid tape, 5-cm Fixomull or Hypafix hypoallergenic tape.

POSITION

Standing with the feet slightly apart and 20° externally rotated. Hands crossed over the shoulders, and the thoracic spine rotated away from the side to be taped.

APPLICATION

Apply the hypoallergenic tape in the same sequence as the rigid tape, as follows:
1. Apply a continuous strip of rigid tape from the anteromedial aspect of the lower third of the thigh, moving superolaterally, behind the greater trochanter, over the SIJ to finish on the contralateral side of the low lumbar spine (Fig. 8.2).
2. Increase tension when passing over the posterolateral aspect, by creating skin folds with the therapist's other hand. This is done by pinching the soft tissue and moving it in the direction opposite to the tape application (Figs 8.3 and 8.4).
3. Apply two closing locks with Fixomull to either end of the tape (Fig. 8.5).

CHECK FUNCTION

Ask the patient to resume a single leg stance. The technique should neutralize any Trendelenberg sign.

CONTRAINDICATION

Ensure that the rigid tape does not extend beyond the hypoallergenic tape, thus avoiding possible skin irritation. Avoid using rigid tape with older patients.

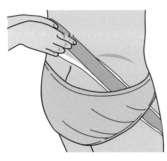

Figure 8.2

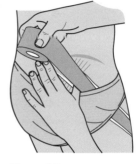

Figure 8.3

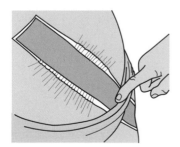

Figure 8.4

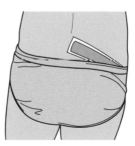

Figure 8.5

Sacroiliac joint

W.A. Hing and D.A. Reid

INDICATION

Pain with weight-bearing and walking. Diagnosed SIJ dysfunction which responds to Mulligan mobilization with movement (MWM). Patients may complain of leg pain mimicking a disc, but with normal straight-leg raise (SLR). Also with positive active straight-leg-raise test (Vleeming).

FUNCTION

Taping corrects the positional fault, by holding the ilium in its correct position on the sacrum. In general, there are two positional faults: (1) anterior innominate, where the ilium will be glided *posterior* to the sacrum; and (2) posterior innominate, where the ilium will be glided *anterior* to the sacrum.

MATERIALS

Spray adhesive or hypoallergenic undertape (Fixomull or Mefix), 3.8-cm strapping tape.

POSITION

If taping for an anterior innominate – patient in prone lying.

APPLICATION

Taping for anterior innonimate – pain with McKenzie extension in lying (Fig. 8.6).
1. Begin with the tape in front of the anterior superior iliac spine. Wrap the tape obliquely and superiorly to terminate over the lumbar spine (Fig. 8.7).
2. Secure with a second piece of tape (Fig. 8.8).

CHECK FUNCTION

Assess original painful movements (i.e. extension in lying, extension in standing, flexion in standing). Movements should now have pain-free full range of motion and function.

CONTRAINDICATION

If taping causes changes or an increase in pain. Tape should not be left on for more than 48 h, and should be removed at any hint of skin irritation.

Figure 8.6

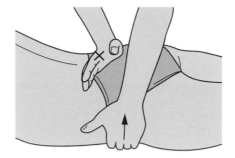

Figure 8.7

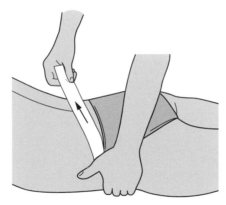

Figure 8.8

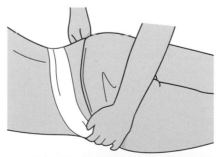

Tips

If the patient has pain with gait, try walking behind the patient, manually applying the MWM posterior glide to the ilium. If this is successful, taping should have positive results.

Chronic low-back and leg pain

J. McConnell

INDICATION

Nerve root irritation.

FUNCTION

Unloads irritated neural and fascial tissue.

MATERIALS

Hypoallergenic tape (Endurafix/Fixomull/Hypafix/Mefix), 3.8-cm tape.

POSITION

Patient standing.

APPLICATION

Apply the hypoallergenic tape to the area to be taped:
1. Anchor the first tape at the ischium and follow the gluteal fold proximal to the greater trochanter, lifting the soft tissue proximally (Fig. 8.9).
2. The second tape is parallel to the natal cleft with the skin lifted towards the buttock. The third tape joins the first and second tapes and runs lateral to medial (Fig. 8.10).
3. The tape then follows the appropriate nerve root and is placed at a diagonal, first on the upper leg and then on the lower leg, with the skin being lifted towards the head each time (Fig. 8.11).

CHECK FUNCTION

Check the painful activity, which should now be pain-free if the tape has been applied properly.

CONTRAINDICATION

Skin allergy – the skin must be protected before taping.

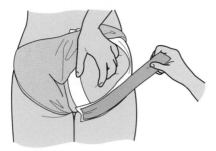

Figure 8.9

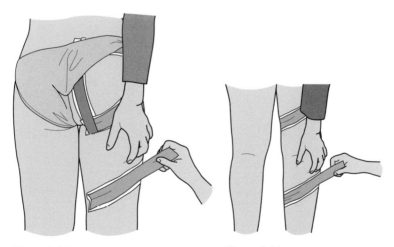

Figure 8.10

Figure 8.11

Tips

The symptoms may intensify slightly distally, but as soon as the distal tape is in situ, the symptoms minimize.

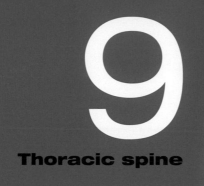

9 chapter ◀◀

Thoracic spine

CHAPTER CONTENTS

Thoracic spine taping

W.A. Hing and D.A. Reid

INDICATION

Thoracic pain and posture correction. Neck pain associated with cervical end-range rotation or neck retraction. Application following Mulligan sustained natural apophyseal glides (SNAGs) to cervicothoracic or thoracic spine.

FUNCTION

Maintains neutral to retracted thoracic posture, and avoids pain-provoking postures. Decreases pain during specific neck movements (end-range cervical rotation or retraction), by holding shoulder girdle into a more retracted position.

MATERIALS

Spray adhesive or hypoallergenic undertape (Fixomull or Mefix), 3.8-cm or 5-cm strapping tape.

POSITION

Patient sitting with shoulders retracted.

APPLICATION

1. Place a single horizontal strip of tape across the shoulder blades of the patient, taping the scapulae into a mid-range, retracted position (Fig. 9.1).
2. The tape should lie just under the spines of the scapulae, running from lateral border to lateral border of each shoulder blade.
3. Place a second piece of tape over the initial taping.

CHECK FUNCTION

Assess original painful movements (i.e. cervical rotation or arm function and ability to reach). Movements should now be pain-free and limited at end of range.

CONTRAINDICATION

If taping causes changes or an increase in pain. Tape should not be left on for more than 48 h, and should be removed at any hint of skin irritation. If there is a potential for tape reaction, use hypoallergenic undertape such as Fixomull.

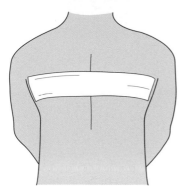

Figure 9.1

Tips

This procedure is easy to apply with the patient in the correct position, so a family member could be taught to do the taping. This would allow the tape to be removed at night and reapplied in the morning, preventing the risk of an adverse skin reaction.

Thoracic spine unload

D. Kneeshaw

INDICATION

Thoracic facet sprain. Overuse of the thoracic paraspinal muscles.

FUNCTION

To support specific vertebrae and reduce muscle activity at that vertebral level.

MATERIALS

Hypoallergenic tape (Fixomull or Mefix), 4-cm rigid strapping tape.

POSITION

Neutral scapula posture.

APPLICATION

1. Using hypoallergenic tape, lay the tape down to form a small square surrounding the offending vertebrae, to about one vertebra above and below.
2. Using rigid tape, attach one end of the tape to a corner of the square and lay the tape to the adjacent corner, shortening the tissue to create a puckering effect (Fig. 9.2).
3. Repeat the previous procedure for each side of the square.

CONTRAINDICATION

Patients with a history of hypersensitive skin.

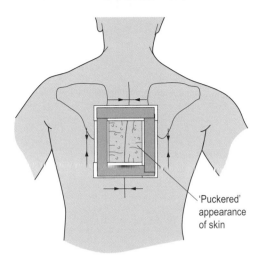

'Puckered'
appearance
of skin

Figure 9.2

Tips

The exposed tissue in the centre of the square should have an orange-peel appearance.
Useful for acute, painful conditions that have an associated muscular spasm.

Winging scapulae

D. Kneeshaw

INDICATION

Instability, impingement, tendinitis.

FUNCTION

To reposition the scapulae to a neutral posture and allow proper activation of the serratus anterior and lower trapezius.

MATERIALS

Hypoallergenic tape (Fixomull or Mefix), 4-cm rigid strapping tape.

POSITION

Retracted and depressed scapular posture.

APPLICATION

1. Using hypoallergenic tape, form an overlapping row of three to four straps from just lateral of the medial border (central) of one scapula to the other.
2. Using rigid tape, apply over the hypoallergenic tape with firm pressure to reinforce the retracted and depressed scapular posture (Fig. 9.3).

CHECK FUNCTION

Assess scapulohumeral rhythm. Assess amount of winging by attempting to push your index finger under the inferior angle of the scapula – only one phalange should be concealed.

CONTRAINDICATION

Patients with a history of hypersensitive skin.

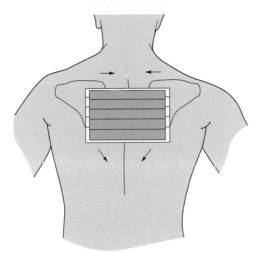

Figure 9.3

Scapular control – Watson's strap

D. Kneeshaw

INDICATION

Impingement, tendinitis.

FUNCTION

To reposition the scapulae in a neutral position and allow proper activation of the rhomboids and trapezius muscles.

MATERIALS

Hypoallergenic tape (Fixomull or Mefix), 4-cm rigid strapping tape.

POSITION

Neutral scapular posture.

APPLICATION

1. Lay the hypoallergenic tape from the axilla, across the middle third of the scapula, to the mid point of the spine of the contralateral scapula.
2. Using rigid tape, begin at the axilla and apply no pressure until the tape meets the lateral border of the scapula.
3. The therapist then places one hand in the axilla and applies a superomedial pressure to the scapula, thus resulting in a lateral rotation movement (Fig. 9.4).
4. Simultaneously apply the tape to the mid point of the spine of the contralateral scapula.

CHECK FUNCTION

Assess scapulohumeral rhythm in abduction and forward flexion. Assess pain levels compared with before.

CONTRAINDICATION

Patients with a history of hypersensitive skin.

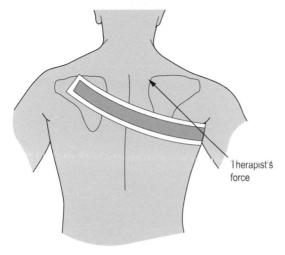

Therapist's force

Figure 9.4

Tips

Ask hirsute individuals to shave their armpits 48 h before tape application.

Scapular retraction

D. Kneeshaw

INDICATION

Instability, impingement, tendinitis.

FUNCTION

Reposition the scapulae to a neutral posture and shorten the rhomboids, lower trapezius or serratus anterior.

MATERIALS

Hypoallergenic tape (Fixomull or Mefix), 4-cm rigid strapping tape.

POSITION

Scapulae in retracted, depressed posture.

APPLICATION

1. Using hypoallergenic tape, lay the tape from the coracoid process posteriorly across the lateral aspect of the acromion to a point just lateral to the T7 spinous process.
2. Using rigid tape, lay over the hypoallergenic tape – without pressure – to the posterior aspect of the shoulder, and finally apply a firm pressure medially to position the scapula in a retracted, depressed posture (Fig. 9.5).

CONTRAINDICATION

Patients with a history of hypersensitive skin.

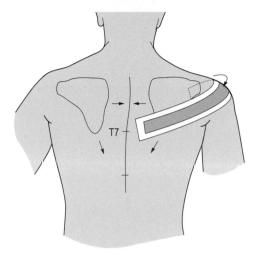

T7

Figure 9.5

Tips

Do not over-retract or depress the scapula.

Serratus anterior taping

U. McCarthy Persson

INDICATION

Scapular dyskinesis or poor upward and downward scapular motion control during shoulder elevation. Altered abnormal scapular rotation can contribute to subscapular impingement.

FUNCTION

To facilitate the action of the serratus anterior muscle to upwardly rotate the scapula during shoulder elevation.

MATERIALS

3.8-cm rigid tape, 5-cm Fixomull or Hypafix hypoallergenic tape.

POSITION

Standing with the arm relaxed by the side in a neutral position.

APPLICATION

1. Apply the hypoallergenic tape without tension from below the nipple around the chest wall through the axilla and over the inferior angle of the scapula. Finish 2 cm lateral to the spine without crossing the midline.
2. Start the rigid tape below the nipple on the hypoallergenic tape. Pull the tape posteriorly around the chest wall. Place the thumb on the inferior scapular angle and push the skin laterally and anteriorly while pulling the tape firmly in a posterior direction over the thumb. The tension applied on the tape should form a vertical skin fold just lateral to the inferior angle of the scapula (Fig 9.6).

CHECK FUNCTION

Assess for improvement in active movement, pain and muscle function. The tape should feel tight but supportive when applied correctly.

CONTRAINDICATION

Ensure that the rigid tape does not extend beyond the hypoallergenic tape, thus avoiding possible skin irritation.

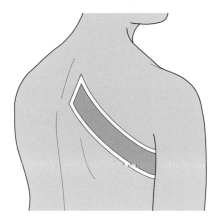

Figure 9.6

10

chapter
◄◄

Shoulder girdle

CHAPTER CONTENTS

Shoulder taping techniques – introduction

D. Morrissey

The following shoulder tapes can be applied either in combination or in isolation. Scapular upward rotation, external rotation, posterior tilt and upper trapezius inhibition can be applied in any combination according to the patient presentation. Shoulder girdle elevation or upward rotation must be applied before acromioclavicular joint congruency taping to ensure the acromium is elevated prior to bringing the clavicle down.

Shoulder girdle elevation

D. Morrissey

INDICATION

Symptom-associated excessive depression of the scapula at rest or during movement, *or* an acromioclavicular (AC) joint asymmetry.

FUNCTION

To elevate the shoulder girdle.

MATERIALS

5-cm Mefix/Hypafix as an underlayer for 4-cm zinc oxide tape.

POSITION

The tape is applied with the shoulder girdle in a relatively elevated position.

APPLICATION

The Mefix is first applied without any tension (Fig. 10.1):
1. Two-thirds of the circumference of the upper arm at a level just below the deltoid tuberosity as an initial anchor strip.
2. From the anterior arm over the anchor strip to the posterior neck just lateral to the spinous process of C7/T1.
3. From the posterior arm over the anchor strip to the anterior neck just lateral to the sternocleidomastoid or the angle of the neck, depending on individual anatomy.

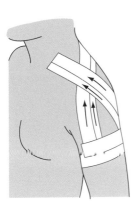

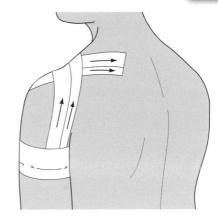

Figure 10.1   **Figure 10.2**

The zinc oxide is then applied with minimal tension (Fig. 10.2):

4. From the anterior arm over the anchor strip to the posterior neck just lateral to the spinous process of C7/T1. This can be repeated, varying the angle of pull.
5. From the posterior arm over the anchor strip to the anterior neck just lateral to the sternocleidomastoid. This can be repeated, varying the angle of pull.
6. Finally a locking strip is applied over the anchor strips.

CHECK FUNCTION

Check that full movement is possible and that the anterior neck area is not excessively stressed by the tape.

CONTRAINDICATION

Allergic reaction, open skin wounds.

INSTRUCTION TO PATIENT

The tape may be left on for up to 3 days providing the skin is not red or itchy. Avoiding excessive wetting, with subsequent hairdryer use, means it will last longer. At least a day should be left before reapplication. Removal must be gradual and gentle.

Acromioclavicular joint congruency

D. Morrissey

INDICATION

This technique is used after satisfactory elevation of the acromium has been achieved with elevation or upward rotation taping, where there is an AC joint asymmetry due to postural factors or trauma.

FUNCTION

To improve the congruency of the AC joint at rest and during movement.

MATERIALS

5-cm Mefix/Hypafix as an underlayer, 4-cm zinc oxide tape.

POSITION

Sitting with the shoulder girdle in a passively elevated position.

APPLICATION

First apply either the *upward rotation* or *elevation taping* procedures as detailed elsewhere. Then apply a strip of tape from the anterior chest wall just below the coracoid over the distal clavicle, up to but not covering the AC joint line, over the scapula and attach onto the rib angles near T9/10. This tape must pass beyond the scapula (Fig. 10.3).

CHECK FUNCTION

Check that full movement is possible and that the anterior neck area is not excessively stressed by the tape.

CONTRAINDICATION

Allergic reaction, open skin wounds, planned surgery.

INSTRUCTION TO PATIENT

The tape may be left on for up to 3 days providing the skin is not red or itchy. At least a day should be left before reapplication. Removal must be gradual and gentle.

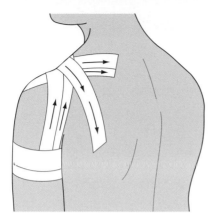

Figure 10.3

Subluxation of acromioclavicular joint

W.A. Hing and D.A. Reid

INDICATION

Disruption of the AC joint complex, grades 1 and 2.

FUNCTION

To provide a degree of support to stretched ligaments.

MATERIALS

Spray adhesive or hypoallergenic undertape (Fixomull or Mefix), 3.8-cm strapping tape, 3.8-cm elastic adhesive bandage (EAB).

POSITION

Patient sitting with the hand on the hip or, alternatively, rest the elbow on a table so the arm sits at about 45° away from the side.

APPLICATION

1. Apply a piece of hypoallergenic undertape (Fixomull) as an anchor from the front of the chest over the end of the clavicle to the shoulder blade.
2. Attach a length of tape from the anchor down the front of the arm, around the elbow and back up the other side of the arm to the anchor on the shoulder blade (Fig. 10.4).
3. Next, apply an EAB in the same fashion. (Adhesive tape can also be used.)
4. Apply an EAB anchor around the arm just above the biceps muscle. Ensure that it is not too tight to compromise the circulation (Fig. 10.5). Reapply an anchor over the AC joint.
5. Once this is secure, cut off the tape which has been previously applied around the elbow (Fig. 10.6). Removing this originally applied piece of tape allows more freedom of movement for the arm. The reason for originally applying it was to create enough tension on the AC joint to keep it down. They often pop up when damaged.

CONTRAINDICATION

Grade 3 injury will probably need orthopaedic review.

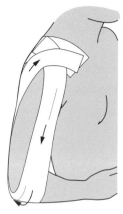

Figure 10.4

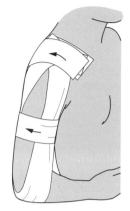

Figure 10.5

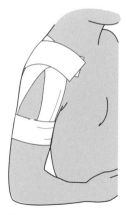

Figure 10.6

Acromioclavicular joint strap

D. Kneeshaw

INDICATION

Ligamentous sprain about the AC joint.

FUNCTION

To reduce superior migration of the clavicle and allow proper rotation and translation of the joint.

MATERIALS

Hypoallergenic tape (Fixomull or Mefix), 4-cm rigid strapping tape.

POSITION

Arm by the side in neutral posture.

APPLICATION

1. Using hypoallergenic tape, lay the tape from around mid-height of the pectoralis major, superior to the nipple, to the inferior angle of the scapula (Fig. 10.7).
2. Using rigid tape, lay the tape from anterior to posterior with firm pressure in an inferior direction, on the posterior side. Do not apply posterior force, only inferior.

CHECK FUNCTION

Assess the amount of AC joint elevation in horizontal flexion and forward flexion. Assess pain levels compared with before.

CONTRAINDICATION

Patients with a history of hypersensitive skin.

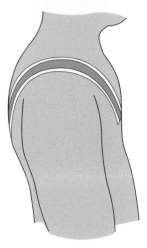

Figure 10.7

Acromioclavicular joint taping

A. Hughes

INDICATION

Acute distraction of the AC joint (grade 1–3 ligamentous injuries). May be modified for glenohumeral joint instability.

FUNCTION

To relieve superior shoulder pain by: (1) maintaining approximation of the acromion and distal end of the clavicle following AC joint injury; and (2) assisting in depressing the distal end of the clavicle.

MATERIALS

5-cm hypoallergenic pretape (Fixomull/Hypafix), 3.8-cm rigid tape, 10-cm elastic adhesive tape.

POSITION

Sitting with the arm supported and abducted 50–60° to the horizontal, and 10° horizontal flexion.

APPLICATION

1. Apply the Fixomull tape in the same sequence as the rigid tape which follows, and ensure that the rigid tape does not extend beyond the border of the Fixomull as skin reaction is likely to occur in this area of the body.
2. Apply two strips of rigid tape from below the inferior angle of the scapula, over the shoulder (avoiding the AC joint) to the subpectoral region. Pull down on the clavicle and gather up the pectoral soft tissues prior to attaching (Fig. 10.8).
3. Apply one to two incomplete anchors to the humerus distal to the deltoid insertion, overlapping by two-thirds.
4. Attach two support strips from the anterior and posterior aspects of the humeral anchors. Passing in a superoposterior and superoanterior direction, attach to the posterior and anterior aspects of the thoracic anchor respectively. Repeat with two more support strips, overlapping the previous strips by two-thirds (Fig. 10.9).
5. Reapply the original anchors on the humerus.
6. Apply two locking anchors to the thorax with either Fixomull or an elastic adhesive tape, to ensure the thoracic tapes do not lift during arm elevation (Figs 10.10 and 10.11).

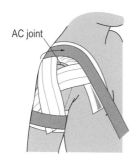

AC joint

Figure 10.8

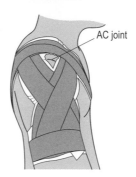

AC joint

Figure 10.9

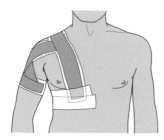

Figure 10.10

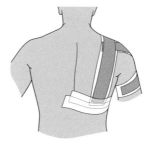

Figure 10.11

CHECK FUNCTION

In a standing position, the affected arm should be maintained in approximately 10° of abduction. Note the freedom of motion available into elevation (Fig. 10.12).

CONTRAINDICATION

Avoid using rigid tape with older patients as skin reaction may occur. In this case, the complete technique may be applied with hypoallergenic tape such as Fixomull/Hypafix.

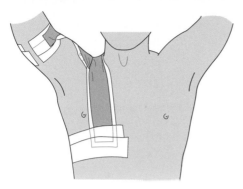

Figure 10.12

Tips

Adapt the technique for glenohumeral joint instabilities by applying the humeral crossover tapes (see Fig. 10.9) to cover a greater area of the anterior glenohumeral joint (limiting horizontal extension) or to the posterior glenohumeral joint (limiting horizontal flexion). This will also restrict elevation of the arm.

The AC joint is not covered by tape with this technique (see Figs 10.8–10.10). It is therefore possible to use therapeutic agents while the tape is in place.

Acromioclavicular taping for sport using stretch tape

O. Rouillon

INDICATION

Return to sport after AC subluxation. Preventive for athletes with residual after-effects. For sprains where rigid tape is not necessary.

FUNCTION

To control the clavicle actively and passively during sport.

MATERIALS

Lubricant, three to four gauze squares, one to two rolls of 6-cm stretch tape, 10-cm cohesive bandage.

POSITION

Sitting with the arm abducted 80°.

APPLICATION

Protect the nipple with lubricant and pad. Protect the AC joint with lubricant and pad. Place an anchor of 6-cm stretch tape around the upper arm in the V of the deltoid without tension. Place a semicircular anchor around the thorax (Fig. 10.13).

Support strips

1. Using 6-cm stretch tape, start the first strip at the sternoclavicular joint and pull with moderate tension over the AC joint to finish on the posterior aspect of the arm anchor (Fig. 10.14).
2. The second strip starts at the base of the neck posteriorly and crosses the AC joint, finishing on the anterior aspect of the arm anchor (Fig. 10.15).
3. The third strip starts on the thoracic vertebra, crosses the AC joint and finishes on the arm anchor anterior to strip 2 (Fig. 10.16).

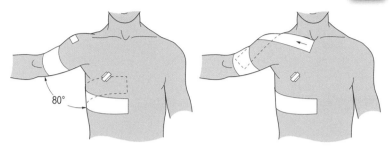

Figure 10.13   **Figure 10.14**

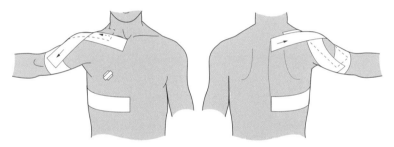

Figure 10.15   **Figure 10.16**

Three more strips are applied (with 6-cm tape):

4. The first strip passes from the posterior thoracic anchor over the AC joint, to finish on the anterior thoracic anchor in the sagittal plane (Fig. 10.17).

5. The second strip starts at a 30° angle to the first and crosses the first strip at the AC joint.

6. The third strip is symmetrical to the second and crosses the previous two strips at the AC joint (Fig. 10.18).

Anchors (locking strips)

Using 6-cm stretch tape, repeat the initial anchors around the arm and thorax (Fig. 10.19). To maintain the tape job in place, apply a 10-cm cohesive bandage a couple of times around the thorax.

CHECK FUNCTION

Test the active range of motion. Check if the tape job is supportive.

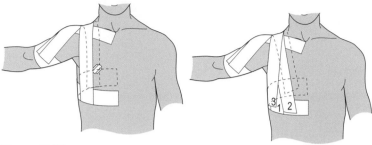

Figure 10.17

Figure 10.18

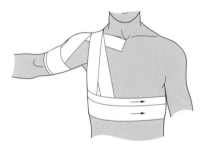

Figure 10.19

Scapular upward rotation

D. Morrissey

INDICATION

This technique is used where scapulohumeral rhythm is compromised, for example in subacromial impingement.

FUNCTION

To proprioceptively facilitate upward rotation of the scapula during arm elevation while the patient is consciously relearning an improved movement pattern.

MATERIALS

10-cm Mefix/Hypafix, 4-cm zinc oxide tape.

POSITION

Patient seated with the arm resting slightly away from the side on a slight 'raise', e.g. roll of tape.

APPLICATION

The tape is applied with the scapula in the 'corrected' or upwardly rotated position, which can be achieved by active positioning taught by the therapist.
1. The Mefix is first applied without tension from just lateral to the thoracic spines of T3–T9 down and laterally to the mid-axillary line. The zinc oxide tape is then applied, either from medial to lateral or visa versa, pushing the inferior angle of the scapula laterally with the thumb and bunching the overlying skin slightly (Fig. 10.20).
2. Three or four strips of zinc oxide tape are applied in this way.

CHECK FUNCTION

Check that full elevation is possible. Take care that axillary hair is not trapped and the soft underarm skin is not excessively tensioned, as this area can easily break down.

CONTRAINDICATION

Allergic reaction, open skin wounds.

INSTRUCTION TO PATIENT

The tape may be left on for up to 3 days providing the skin is not red or itchy. At least a day should be left before reapplication. Removal must be gradual and gentle.

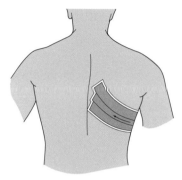

Figure 10.20

Relocation of the humeral head

J. McConnell

INDICATION

Anterior shoulder instability, impingement problems, rotator cuff tears and adhesive capsulitis.

FUNCTION

Taping corrects the positional fault by lifting the anterior aspect of the humeral head up and back, to increase the space between the humeral head and the acromium.

MATERIALS

Hypoallergenic tape (Endurafix/Fixomull/Hypafix/Mefix), 3.8-cm tape.

POSITION

Patient standing or sitting on a chair or stool, arms resting by the side.

APPLICATION

Apply the hypoallergenic tape to the area to be taped.
1. Anchor a strip of tape on the anterior aspect of the glenohumeral joint.
2. With the thumb of the other hand, lift the head of the humerus up and back (Fig. 10.21).
3. Firmly pull the tape diagonally across the scapula, to finish just medial to the inferior border of the scapula.

Care must be taken not to pull too hard on the skin anteriorly, as the skin is sensitive in this region and may break down if not looked after properly.

CHECK FUNCTION

Check painful activity, which should now be pain-free if the tape has been applied properly.

CONTRAINDICATION

Skin allergy – the skin must be protected before taping.

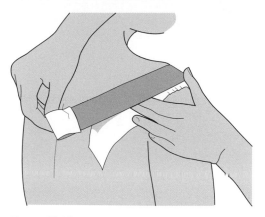

Figure 10.21

Tips

To ensure long-term reductions in symptoms, work on improving thoracic spine mobility and muscle training of the scapular and glenohumeral stabilizers.

Multidirectional instability

J. McConnell

INDICATION

Multidirectional shoulder instability.

FUNCTION

Taping stabilizes the head of the humerus in the glenoid cavity.

MATERIALS

Hypoallergenic tape (Endurafix/Fixomull/Hypafix/Mefix), 3.8-cm tape.

POSITION

Patient sitting on a chair or stool, forearm supported on a table at 30° of scaption.

APPLICATION

Apply the hypoallergenic tape to the area to be taped.
1. Anchor the first piece of tape over the middle deltoid and lift the head of the humerus up.
2. The second piece commences anteriorly on the humerus and passes in a diagonal over the clavicle and anchors on the spine of the scapula. The humerus again is lifted superiorly (Fig. 10.22).
3. The third piece of tape is commenced on the posterior deltoid and runs along the spine of the scapula to the nape of the neck. The humerus is lifted superiorly. This piece gives the patient some posterior stability. Without this piece of tape, the patient often feels insecure.

CHECK FUNCTION

Check painful activity, which should now be pain-free if the tape has been applied properly.

CONTRAINDICATION

Skin allergy – the skin must be protected before taping.

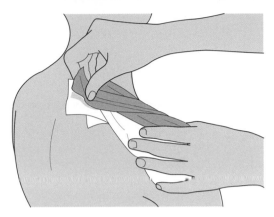

Figure 10.22

Tips

Initially work on training the deltoid muscle as a stabilizer.

Upper trapezius inhibition

D. Morrissey

INDICATION

This technique is used when the upper trapezius muscle is judged to be overactive, with reduction of that overactivity clinically desirable.

FUNCTION

To compress the upper trapezius muscle belly and reduce activity.

MATERIALS

5-cm Mefix/Hypafix as an underlayer for 4-cm zinc oxide tape.

POSITION

Applied with the upper trapezius at rest, arm by the side in a supported position.

APPLICATION

The Mefix is applied first without any tension, as follows:
1. From just over the mid clavicle, with the medial border of the tape adjacent to the angle of the neck (Fig. 10.23).
2. Over the shoulder and attaching as far down as T9/10 on the posterior torso (Fig. 10.24).

The zinc oxide is then applied with minimal tension:
3. From just above the clavicle, attached as far as the middle of the muscle belly from where a strong compressive force is applied to the muscle, and the tail of the tape attached as far down as T9/10.
4. A second strip is rarely required.

CHECK FUNCTION

Check that full movement is possible and the anterior clavipectoral area is not stressed by the tape. The skin can easily break down over a 24-h period.

CONTRAINDICATION

Allergic reaction, open skin wounds.

INSTRUCTION TO PATIENT

The tape may be left on for up to 3 days providing the skin is not red or itchy. Avoiding excessive wetting, with subsequent hairdryer use, means it will last longer. At least a day should be left before reapplication. Removal must be gradual and gentle.

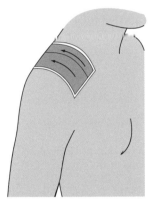

Figure 10.23

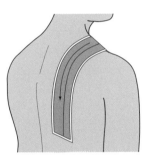

Figure 10.24

Scapular external rotation

D. Morrissey

INDICATION

This technique is used in the situation where excessive scapular internal rotation is associated with symptoms, e.g. shoulder impingement.

FUNCTION

To proprioceptively facilitate external rotation of the scapula during arm elevation while the patient is consciously relearning an improved movement pattern.

MATERIALS

5-cm Mefix/Hypafix as an underlayer for 4-cm zinc oxide tape.

POSITION

The tape is applied with the scapula in the 'corrected' or externally rotated position. This can be achieved by active positioning taught by the therapist, even if it briefly involves suboptimal patterns of muscle activation. Alternatively, passive positioning can be used when the zinc oxide tape is applied.

APPLICATION

1. The Mefix is first applied without any tension from 2 cm proximal to the anterior glenohumeral joint line, around the deltoid just below the acromion to an end position over the ipsilateral T7.
2. The zinc oxide tape is then applied from the anterior glenohumeral joint line to the same end position. It must cross the scapula fully. No more than a little tension on the tape is advised, as the aim is for the tape to apply a pull when the patient loses an optimal position (Figs 10.25 and 10.26).

CHECK FUNCTION

Check that elevation is possible. The only significant (>15%) restriction should be horizontal flexion.

CONTRAINDICATION

Allergic reaction, open skin wounds.

INSTRUCTION TO PATIENT

The patient can leave the tape on for up to 3 days providing the skin is not red or itchy. Avoiding excessive wetting, with subsequent hairdryer use, means it will last longer. At least a day should be left before reapplication. Removal must be gradual and gentle.

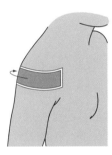

Figure 10.25

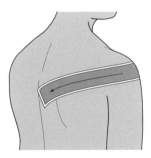

Figure 10.26

Scapular posterior tilt

D. Morrissey

INDICATION

This technique is used when excessive anterior tilt during elevation is noted as being part of the patient's presentation.

FUNCTION

To proprioceptively facilitate posterior rotation of the scapula during arm elevation while the patient is consciously relearning an improved movement pattern.

MATERIALS

5-cm Mefix/Hypafix as an underlayer for 4-cm zinc oxide tape.

POSITION

The tape is applied with the scapula in the 'corrected' or posteriorly rotated position. This can be achieved by active positioning taught by the therapist, even if it briefly involves suboptimal patterns of muscle activation. Alternatively, passive positioning can be used when the zinc oxide tape is applied.

APPLICATION

1. The Mefix is first applied without any tension from 2 cm medial and over the lower end of the anterior glenohumeral joint line, over the clavicle to an end position over the ipsilateral T10.
2. The zinc oxide tape is then applied from the anterior glenohumeral joint line to the same end position. It must cross the scapula fully. No more than a little tension on the tape is advised, as the aim is for the tape to apply a pull when the patient loses an optimal position (Figs 10.27 and 10.28).

CHECK FUNCTION

Check that full elevation is possible. The only significant (>15%) restriction should be extension. Take great care that the soft anterior clavipectoral skin is not under excessive tension as this area can easily break down.

CONTRAINDICATION

Allergic reaction, open skin wounds.

INSTRUCTION TO PATIENT

The tape may be left on for up to 3 days providing the skin is not red or itchy. Avoiding excessive wetting, with subsequent hairdryer use, means it will last longer. At least a day should be left before reapplication. Removal must be gradual and gentle.

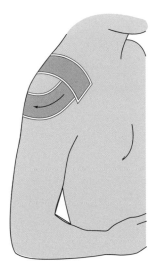

Figure 10.27

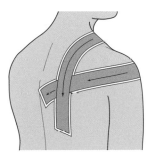

Figure 10.28

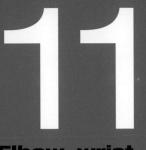

11 chapter ◀◀

Elbow, wrist and hand

CHAPTER CONTENTS

Tennis elbow (lateral epicondylosis)

W.A. Hing and D.A. Reid

INDICATION

Lateral epicondyle pain.

FUNCTION

To reduce the loading on the extensor mechanism, especially in movements of the forearm and wrist involving gripping and pronation.

MATERIALS

Spray adhesive or hypoallergenic undertape (Fixomull or Mefix), 3.8-cm strapping tape, shaver.

POSITION

Patient sitting or standing with the elbow flexed to 90° and the forearm fully supinated.

APPLICATION

1. Place an anchor midway around the forearm (Fig. 11.1).
2. With the arm in the above position, attach a strip of tape to the anchor on the medial side of the forearm. Direct it obliquely up the arm to slightly above the lateral epicondyle. Continue the tape around the lateral part of the triceps and finish on the medial aspect of the biceps (Fig. 11.2).
3. Apply a second strip of tape, following the same lines and overlapping the first strip by a third, usually in a more lateral direction (Fig. 11.3).
4. Reapply the first anchor.

CHECK FUNCTION

Once complete, the patient should feel the tape restrict the movements of elbow extension and pronation.

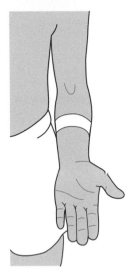

Figure 11.1

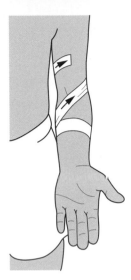

Figure 11.2

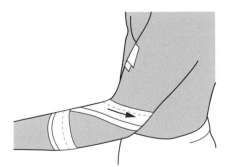

Figure 11.3

Simple epicondylitis technique

R. Macdonald

INDICATION

Tennis elbow – inflammation at the origin of the extensor tendons.

FUNCTION

To relieve stress on the origin of the tendon attachments. To realign the pull of the extensor tendons.

MATERIALS

3.8-cm tape (with strong adhesive mass), 5-cm cohesive bandage.

POSITION

Patient standing and facing the operator with pronated arm resting on the chair back.

APPLICATION

1. Visually observe the contracted belly of the extensor carpi radialis brevis muscle, by applying resistance to the patient's extension of the third and fourth finger and wrist.
2. The patient flexes the elbow 90° across the chest to rest lightly on the opposite forearm. Take a strip of tape 10–15 cm long.
3. Stick the tape to the midline (palmar aspect) of the forearm just distal to the elbow crease, and spiral it superolaterally over the lateral epicondyle, to the olecranon/posteroinferior aspect of the humerus (Fig. 11.4).
4. Before attaching the tape, place the thumb of your other hand under the belly of the muscle and draw the tape firmly across the soft tissues to form a fold (Fig. 11.5).
5. Repeat this strip once more proximally, if necessary.

Hold in place with one or two turns of a cohesive bandage in a figure-of-eight pattern.

CHECK FUNCTION

Ask the patient to make a fist to see if the technique is supportive and relieves stress on the epicondyle.

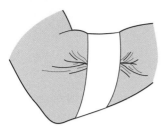

Figure 11.4

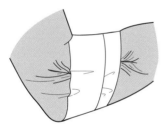

Figure 11.5

Tips

Teach the technique to a friend or family member, as it is easy to apply.

Elbow hyperextension sprain

R. Macdonald

INDICATION

Elbow hyperextension, impingement, sprained medial collateral ligament.

FUNCTION

To limit the degree of elbow extension.

MATERIALS

Adhesive spray, gauze square, 7.5-cm stretch tape, 3.8-cm and 2.5-cm tape, 5-cm cohesive bandage.

POSITION

Patient standing, facing operator with the supinated flexed forearm resting on the back of the chair (with the fist clenched for application of anchors).

APPLICATION

Spray the arm, and apply a lubricated gauze square to the cubital fossa. Apply an anchor of stretch tape around the belly of the biceps (contracted), and another around the proximal third of the forearm.

1. Flex elbow 45–60° and measure the distance between the upper and lower anchors.
2. Taking five strips of 2.5-cm tape (this length), construct a check rein (fan) on the table.
3. Apply one end of the fan to the distal anchor and secure it in place with two or three strips of tape on front of the arm only. Before attaching the other end to the proximal anchor, test the range of motion manually, making sure that full extension is blocked by at least 2° (remember that skin on the upper arm is very mobile).
4. Reapply original anchors to lock down the ends (Fig. 11.6). Spiral up the arm with a cohesive bandage as far as the axilla to prevent skin drag. Secure the end with a strip of tape.

CHECK FUNCTION

Can the patient hold a racket comfortably, and swing forehand/backhand with confidence?

CONTRAINDICATION

Skin allergy or friable skin.

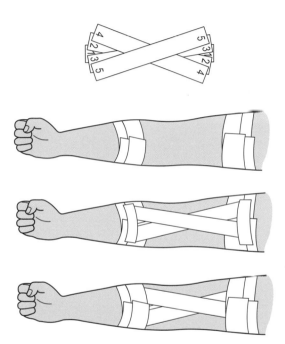

Figure 11.6

> **Tips**
>
> The check rein is very useful for blocking range of motion at many joints – wrist (flexion/extension, radial/ulnar deviation), ankle, knee (genu recurvatum).

Prophylactic wrist taping

D. Reese

INDICATION

Prevention of injuries by wrist extension in sport, e.g. in gymnastics, strength training and others.

FUNCTION

To reduce wrist extension by applying material over the dorsal aspect of the wrist, without causing circulation restriction and carpal tunnel problems often associated with supporting the wrist.

MATERIALS

2.5-cm or 3.75-cm tape, depending on the size of the wrist. A small piece of foam rubber, shaped to cover the palmar aspect of the wrist.

POSITION

Patient standing or sitting while making a fist.

APPLICATION

The patient should be clean, dry and shaved on the area to be taped. Start by having the patient actively make a fist. Place a spongy foam rubber square on the palmar side of the wrist to protect the tendons (Fig. 11.7).

Anchors

Anchors 1, 2 and 3 should be placed starting approximately 5 cm proximal to the ulnar and radial styloid (Fig. 11.8). Apply the tape so that it conforms to the natural angle of the lower arm and hand junction. Overlap distally approximately one-third of the width of the first anchor. The bottom part of the last anchor should lie forward to the base of the second to fifth metacarpals. Check to see that the anchors do not constrict the range of motion.

Support

The support should cover the entire dorsal aspect of the wrist from the styloid processes to the base of the second to fifth metacarpals. The tape is taken back and forth over the area but never circular. The amount is dependent on the amount of support required. Five to six overlaps are common (Fig. 11.9).

Anchor lock

Anchors 1, 2 and 3 should be placed covering the first three (Fig. 11.10).

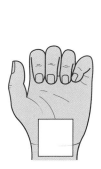

Figure 11.7

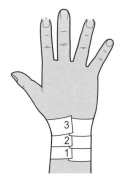

Figure 11.8

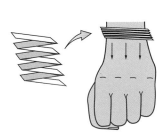

Figure 11.9

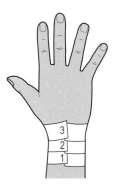

Figure 11.10

CHECK FUNCTION

Is the wrist support adequate for the manoeuvre? If not, adjust by applying more material over the dorsal aspect of the wrist. Check action.

CONTRAINDICATION

Circulation problems to the hand can occur if proper application is not followed. This taping is to be used only when the patient is active.

Notes

The anchors alone, applied as described above, may be used as a simple wrist taping for strength.

Tips

Best applied directly to the skin dorsally.

Wrist taping

K.E. Wright

INDICATION

Sprains and strains to the wrist.

FUNCTION

To provide support and stability for the wrist.

MATERIALS

3.8-cm adhesive tape, 7.5-cm elastic tape.

POSITION

For hyperextension injuries, position the wrist in slight flexion and fingers spread apart. For hyperflexion injuries, position the wrist in slight extension and fingers spread apart.

APPLICATION

1. Apply an anchor strip of 3.8-cm adhesive tape around the mid forearm.
2. Using 7.5-cm elastic tape, cut a strip 30–40 cm in length. In the middle of the tape strip, cut two small holes, approximately 2.5 cm from each side of the tape (Fig. 11.11). With full tension applied to the tape, place the third and fourth phalanges through the cut-outs (Fig. 11.12). Attach the ends of the elastic tape to the mid-forearm anchor (Fig. 11.13).
3. Secure the procedure by applying an anchor of 3.8-cm adhesive tape over the tape ends (Fig. 11.14).

Figure 11.11

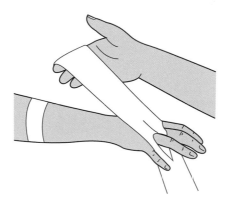

Figure 11.12

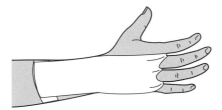

Figure 11.13

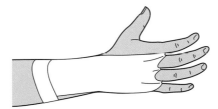

Figure 11.14

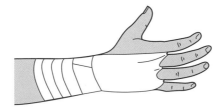

Wrist taping

H. Millson

INDICATION

This is excellent for prevention and treatment of 'paddlers' wrist', i.e. acute tenosynovitis of the forearm. Any wrist pain due to activities of daily living, e.g. overuse of a computer, or diverse sports such as wrestling, rugby, cricket, tennis, badminton, etc.

FUNCTION

To support the wrist and reduce hyperflexion.

MATERIALS

Friars' Balsam or hypoallergenic undertape, 2.5-cm and 5-cm elastic adhesive bandage (EAB).

POSITION

Patient sitting comfortably with the forearm resting, the wrist and fingers in a good functional anatomical position, i.e. slight extension of the wrist (15–20°) and the fingers in slight flexion.

APPLICATION

1. Place an anchor of 5-cm EAB around the mid forearm.
2. Prepare three strips of 2.5-cm tape ahead of time. Cut a V notch at one end of each of the 2.5-cm strips (Fig. 11.15). The length of the tape should go from the palmar surface of the hand below the metacarpophalangeal joints to the mid forearm.
3. These strappings are placed between the fingers over the dorsum of the hand (Fig. 11.16) to the forearm anchor dorsally (Fig. 11.17).
4. Using the 2.5-cm strap, start on the mid-forearm anchor *at the thumb side of the wrist* and go across the wrist, the back of the hand and around the palm at the base of the fingers. This will hold the initial straps down. Do not pull tight. The strapping then goes on around the back of the hand. It crosses itself at the wrist and ends on the anchor on the lateral side of the wrist (Fig. 11.18).

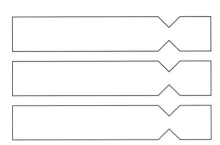

Figure 11.15

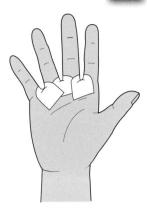

Figure 11.16

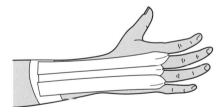

Figure 11.17

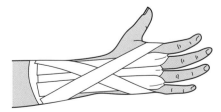

Figure 11.18

5. Three to four more similar straps may be applied, overlapping each other (Figs 11.19 and 11.20).

6. Complete the strapping by closing with 5-cm EAB around the forearm and wrist. This is lightly applied and closed with a small strip of rigid tape to hold the edges together (Fig. 11.21).

CHECK FUNCTION

The strapping must be specific to the function required and must not be restrictive in any way. It is most important that the 2.5-cm straps do not extend a long way into the palm. This could interfere with function. It is vital that the 2.5-cm straps that come around the palmar aspect of the hand hold the three finger straps down adequately in order to stop them pulling out and thus being ineffective.

Caution: Do not pull the straps tight at any point. It is a case of *placing* all the straps on.

CONTRAINDICATION

Any skin allergies, any pain after taping.

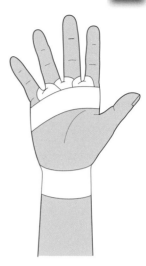

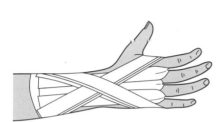

Figure 11.19

Figure 11.20

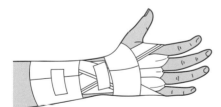

Figure 11.21

Wrist taping

R. Macdonald

INDICATION

Wrist hyperextension, hyperflexion injury.

FUNCTION

To support and limit range of motion.

MATERIALS

Adhesive spray, gauze pad, 3.8-cm and 2.5-cm tape, cohesive bandage.

POSITION

The hand is placed in the open position for anchors, facing the operator.

APPLICATION

Spray the hand and wrist. Apply the pad to the palmar aspect of the wrist, to protect tendons.

Anchors

1. Using 3.8-cm tape, apply either a diagonal anchor across the hand and around the wrist, or an anchor around the middle of the hand. Apply two anchors around the mid forearm below the muscle bulk (Fig. 11.22). With the hand in a slightly flexed position, measure the distance between the proximal and hand anchors.

Check rein

2. Using 2-cm or 2.5-cm tape, construct the check rein (fan) on the table (Fig. 11.23), with five or seven strips, overlapping each strip by half.
3. Apply the fan to the hand anchor first and lock in place. Check the range of motion of the wrist joint, blocking full extension/flexion. Apply the other end to the forearm anchor. Remember that the skin on the forearm is very mobile.

Lock strips

4. Apply strips across the ends of the fan to hold in place, then reapply the original anchors (Fig. 11.24). When applying tape: for hyperextension, slightly flex the wrist; for hyperflexion, slightly extend the wrist.

CHECK FUNCTION

Is pronation/supination restricted? Can the patient hold the racket/bat?

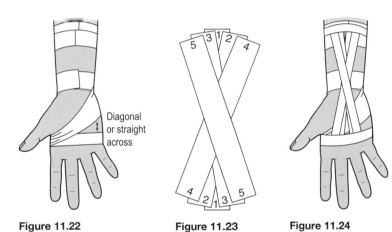

Diagonal or straight across

Figure 11.22   **Figure 11.23**   **Figure 11.24**

Tips

Wrap the hand and wrist with a flesh-coloured cohesive bandage.

Inferior radioulnar joint taping

W.A. Hing and D.A. Reid

INDICATION

Wrist pain, especially with supination or pronation of the wrist. Post-Colles' fracture and conditions in which mobilizations with movement (MWMs) are pain-free and successful.

FUNCTION

Repositions or corrects a positional fault of the ulna in relation to the radius.

MATERIALS

Spray adhesive or hypoallergenic undertape (Fixomull or Mefix), 3.8-cm strapping tape.

POSITION

Patient sitting or standing with arm relaxed and wrist in neutral position.

APPLICATION

Taping if a dorsal glide of the ulna on the radius corrects painful movement.
1. Place tape over the palmar surface of the ulna. Apply and maintain a MWM to the ulna (Fig. 11.25).
2. In a dorsal direction, wrap the tape obliquely across the wrist and around the radius (Fig. 11.26).
3. The tape will end on the palmar aspect of the wrist, near where the taping began.
4. Place a second piece of tape on the initial taping to secure.

CHECK FUNCTION

Ensure there is full range of motion at the wrist. Assess original painful movements (wrist pronation and supination). Movements should now have pain-free full range of motion and function.

CONTRAINDICATION

If taping causes changes, or an increase, in pain. Tape should not be left on for more than 48 h, and should be removed at any hint of skin irritation.

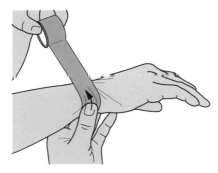

Figure 11.25

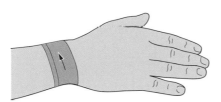

Figure 11.26

Tips

This procedure is easy to apply with the patient in the correct position, so a family member could be taught to do the taping. This would allow the tape to be removed at night and reapplied in the morning, preventing the risk of an adverse skin reaction.

Contusion to the hand

K.E. Wright

INDICATION

Contusion to the hand.

FUNCTION

To provide protection to the bruised hand.

MATERIALS

2.5-cm and 1.25-cm adhesive tape, 5-cm elastic tape, felt or foam pad.

POSITION

Hand palmar aspect down and phalanges abducted.

APPLICATION

1. Cut the foam pad before beginning your procedure.
2. Apply an anchor strip of 2.5-cm adhesive tape around the wrist. Start at the ulnar condyle, cross the dorsal aspect of the distal forearm and encircle the wrist (Fig. 11.27). The foam pad is then applied over the affected area of the hand.
3. Apply strips of 1.25-cm tape. Start on the palmar aspect of the anchor strip, cross between the phalanges and end on the dorsal aspect of the anchor strip (Fig. 11.28). Three strips are applied, between the second and third, third and fourth, and fourth and fifth phalanges (Fig. 11.29).
4. Next, apply a strip of 2.5-cm adhesive tape in a figure-of-eight pattern (Fig. 11.30). Begin on the wrist's dorsal aspect near the ulnar condyle; cross diagonally to the second metacarpal, encircling the distal aspect of the second to fifth metacarpals (Fig. 11.31). Continue across the palmar aspect to the fifth metacarpal, crossing diagonally from here to the radial aspect of the wrist and encircle the wrist (Fig. 11.32). Two to three figure-of-eights can be applied.
5. This technique is completed with a second anchor strip of 2.5-cm adhesive tape applied around the wrist. A continuous figure-of-eight strip of 5-cm elastic tape is applied to give additional support (Fig. 11.33).

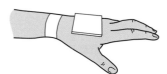

Figure 11.27

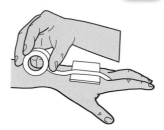

Figure 11.28

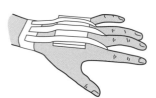

Figure 11.29

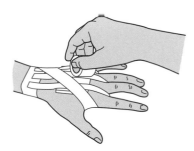

Figure 11.30

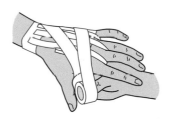

Figure 11.31

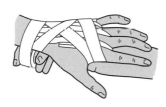

Figure 11.32

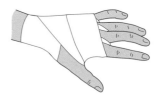

Figure 11.33

Palm protective taping (the Russell web)

C. Armstrong

INDICATION

Unconditioned/uncalloused palms in gymnastics.

FUNCTION

To act as a layer of protection over the skin on the palm of the hand. To help the patient maintain a grip on gymnastic apparatus.

MATERIALS

Adhesive spray, lubricant, 10-cm or 7.5-cm stretch tape, 3.75-cm tape.

POSITION

Patient standing with the arm held forwards and palm up.

APPLICATION

1. Shave the wrist.
2. Lubricate the web space between the fingers and apply gauze (Fig. 11.34).
3. Apply adhesive spray to the hand, including the wrist.
4. Using a length of 10-cm stretch tape that stretches to twice the length of the hand, attach the tape to the base of the hand so that the hand is in the middle of the length of tape (Fig. 11.35).
5. Starting at the finger end of the tape, make four longitudinal cuts into the tape so that, when stretched, the tape strands fit between the fingers but the unsplit portion covers the palm (Fig. 11.36a).
6. Bring these taut strips up from the palmar aspect of the hand to go on the outside of the index finger on the one side and the little finger on the other. The middle strips come up into the web spaces between each of the fingers. These strips should run down the back of the hand, across the wrist, ending on the back of the distal forearm at the wrist (Fig. 11.36b).

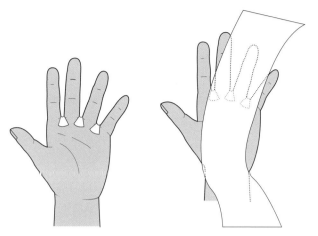

Figure 11.34　　　　**Figure 11.35**

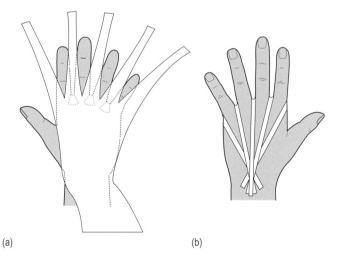

(a)　　　　　　　　　　　　　(b)

Figure 11.36

7. Then, going to the wrist end of the length of tape, cut it down the middle, allowing the cut to correspond to the distal wrist crease. The two strips should be stretched and run around the wrist, anchoring the strands that come along the dorsum of the hand to the wrist (Fig. 11.37a).

8. Cover the wrist strips with 3.75-cm tape (Fig. 11.37b).

CHECK FUNCTION

The patient should be able to flex and extend the wrist without undue discomfort from the tape cutting into the web space between the fingers. The tape should be sufficiently taut not to allow any bunching.

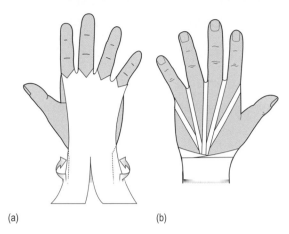

(a)   (b)

Figure 11.37

Tips

On a smaller hand, one might be well advised to use 7.5-cm rather than 10-cm stretch tape.

Protection of the metacarpophalangeal joints for boxers

R. Macdonald

INDICATION

To protect the metacarpophalangeal joints for boxers when training, and in combat sports.

FUNCTION

To maintain the protective padding in place. To leave the palm free for gripping in martial arts.

MATERIALS

2.5-cm and 5-cm stretch tape, adhesive spray, padding/Professional Protective Technology (PPT)/poron or rubber.

APPLICATION

1. Spray the dorsum of the hand and wrist. Cut a protective pad to fit over the four metacarpophalangeal joints. Stick the pad in place and anchor it with 5-cm stretch tape. Apply a 5-cm stretch tape anchor around the wrist (Fig. 11.38).
2. Using 2.5-cm stretch tape, cut four strips long enough to encircle each finger, and anchor on the proximal end of the wrist anchor.
3. The centre of the first strip is placed around the index finger. Cross the two ends over the metacarpophalangeal joint. One winds over the metacarpal of the thumb to attach to the anterior aspect of the wrist anchor. The other end is attached to the wrist anchor, on the dorsum (Fig. 11.39).
4. Repeat this on the middle and ring fingers. Finger 5 is the same as the index finger, with one strip winding around to the palmar aspect of the wrist anchor (Fig. 11.40).

Lock strips

Reapply the wrist anchor and close off with the tape (Fig. 11.41).

CHECK FUNCTION

Can the athlete make a fist without discomfort? Is the pad in the right position for full protection?

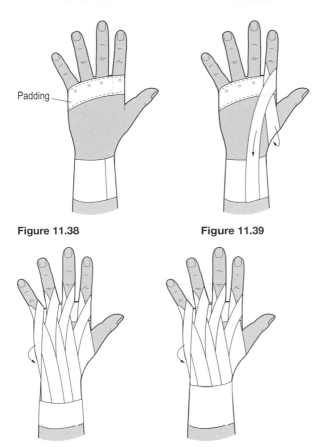

Padding

Figure 11.38   **Figure 11.39**

Figure 11.40   **Figure 11.41**

Notes

The pad may be bevelled to overlay the web of the fingers or lubricated gauze pads may be applied between the fingers.

Tips

Apply adhesive spray directly to the pad. Let it get tacky before sticking it to the metacarpophalangeal joints. If secure, the anchor may not be necessary.

12

chapter ◄◄

Fingers and thumb

CHAPTER CONTENTS

Sprained fingers – buddy system

R. Macdonald

INDICATION

Minor trauma to a finger on the field of play, a ball hitting an extended finger, a jammed finger.

FUNCTION

To protect and support the finger by taping it to its neighbour (functional splint).

MATERIALS

Foam or felt padding, 2.5-cm tape.

POSITION

Standing, facing the operator with the hand outstretched, and the fingers held slightly apart.

APPLICATION

1. Place a strip of felt, foam or cotton wool between the injured finger and the adjacent fingers.
2. Apply strips of tape around the proximal and middle phalanges, with the closures on the dorsal aspect.
3. Do not cover the joint lines with tape.
4. Two or three fingers may be taped together, depending on the sport (Fig. 12.1).

CHECK FUNCTION

Can the patient hold equipment, grasp, throw and catch?

CONTRAINDICATION

Suspected fracture, ligament tear or tendon avulsion.

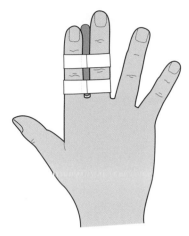

Figure 12.1

Tips

Tape may be ripped down the centre for a small finger.

Single-finger taping

J. O'Neill

FUNCTION

To help support the collateral ligaments of the fingers.

MATERIALS

Tape adherent, 1.25-cm porous tape.

POSITION

The athlete's injured finger is extended in a relaxed position.

APPLICATION

This technique is similar to taping of a collateral ligament sprain of a knee.
1. Apply tape adherent.
2. Apply a 1.25-cm anchor strip around the middle and proximal phalanx (Fig. 12.2).
3. Eight strips of 1.25-cm tape approximately 5–8 cm long are precut and then applied as indicated in Figure 12.3.
4. Place a 2.5-cm strip to cover the tape around the middle and proximal phalanx (Fig. 12.4).
5. Finally, 'buddy tape' the injured finger to the adjacent finger to aid in support (Fig. 12.5).

CHECK FUNCTION

Be watchful of overtightness of the tape.

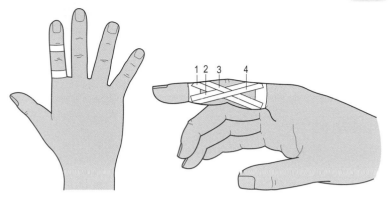

Figure 12.2   Figure 12.3

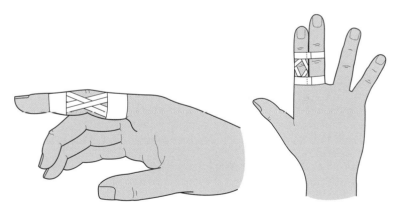

Figure 12.4   Figure 12.5

Tips

When taping fingers, place in about 15° of flexion. This will allow the athlete to feel more comfortable.

Finger joint support

R. Macdonald

INDICATION

Collateral ligament sprain.

FUNCTION

To support the joint in a functional position, allowing flexion and extension of the digits.

MATERIALS

2.5-cm tape, which may be ripped down the centre for a small finger.

POSITION

Patient facing the operator, hand in prone position with the fingers held apart.

APPLICATION

1. Cover the finger nail with a small piece of tape, sticky sides folded together by two-thirds. Stick on just above the nail (Fig. 12.6).
2. Measure the finger from the metacarpophalangeal joint to the finger tip, and rip four strips.
3. Lay one strip diagonally across the proximal interphalangeal joint and wrap the ends around the proximal and distal phalanges (see Fig. 12.6).
4. Repeat on the other side of the joint.
5. Apply these same strips twice more, making sure that the tape does not cover the joint line (Fig. 12.7).
6. Secure the tape with proximal and distal anchors.

CHECK FUNCTION

Can the patient use the finger normally?

CONTRAINDICATION

Suspected fracture, joint disruption or tendon avulsion.

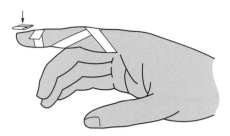

Figure 12.6

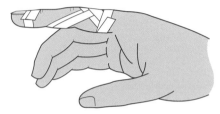

Figure 12.7

Tips

Cover with a finger stall or cohesive bandage if going in water.
A glove may be worn with this technique.

Climber's finger injury

R. Macdonald

INDICATION

Finger flexor tendon strain in climbers, usually the fourth or ring finger.

FUNCTION

Stabilizes the finger in a flexed position and limits extension of the proximal interphalangeal joint.

MATERIALS

2.5-cm rigid tape, 2.5-cm adhesive bandage.

POSITION

Patient sitting with the supinated forearm resting on a table and the hand over the edge, with the finger flexed.

APPLICATION

1. Take about a 15-cm length of tape.
2. Split one end and wrap around the proximal phalanx from the palmar aspect; apply an anchor with the closure on the dorsal aspect.
3. Roll the tape between thumb and index finger to form a rope (Fig. 12.8).
4. Split the other end of the tape and wrap around the middle or distal phalanx (depending on which tendon is strained) to maintain the finger in the flexed position (Fig. 12.9).
5. Place another anchor around the distal phalanx with closure on the dorsal aspect.
6. Wrap the finger with cohesive bandage.

CHECK FUNCTION

Check that the phalanx is held in the flexed position and is stable. Check the circulation.

CONTRAINDICATION

Do not place tape on the nail as it may damage the nail bed on removal.

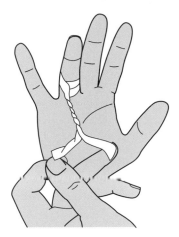

Figure 12.8

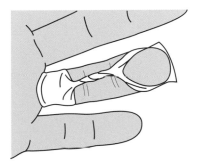

Figure 12.9

Tips

Prior to taping, cover the nail with a small piece of tape folded sticky sides together, with a little bit of the adhesive mass free to stick on the finger proximal to the nail.

Prophylactic thumb taping

D. Reese

INDICATION

Prevention of injuries caused by hyperextension of the thumb in sports, e.g. ice hockey, European handball, skiing, soccer goalkeepers.

FUNCTION

To prevent hyperextension of the thumb and further damage to the volar ligament without inhibiting any other of the vital functions of the thumb. Its simplicity allows the athlete to regulate the tension at any time for better function.

MATERIALS

2.5-cm or 1.25-cm tape stripped (less than the width of the thumb). A small piece of foam rubber shaped to cover the palmar aspect of the wrist.

POSITION

Patient standing or sitting.

APPLICATION

The hand should be clean, dry and shaved in the area to be taped. Start by having the patient actively make a fist. Place a spongy foam rubber square on the palmar side of the wrist to protect the wrist tendons (Fig. 12.10).

Anchors

Anchors 1 and 2 should be placed starting approximately 5 cm proximal to the ulnar and radial styloid. Apply the tape so that it conforms to the natural angle of the lower arm and hand junction. Overlap distally approximately one-third of the width of the first anchor. Check to see that the anchors do not constrict the range of motion (Fig. 12.11).

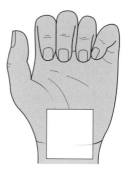

Figure 12.10

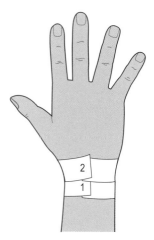

Figure 12.11

Support

Place two strips 60 cm in length that are a little less than the width of the thumb on top of each other. Open the hand and start the support at the base of the first phalanx on the dorsal side of the hand. Pull the tape through the middle line of the thumb, over the thumb nail and over the volar ligament towards the ulnar styloid on the palmar side of the hand (Figs 12.12 and 12.13). Wrap the rest of the support around the wrist (Fig. 12.14).

Lock strip

Lock a small strip around the second phalanx of the thumb as well as a couple of strips on top of each other over the base of the first phalanx (Fig. 12.15).

CHECK FUNCTION

Allow the patient to decide the tension and restriction of the tape that will be used in the activity. Have on hand the equipment or ball for final adjustment.

CONTRAINDICATION

Hypermobility in hyperextension of the thumb.

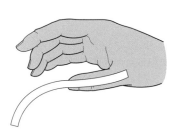

Figure 12.12

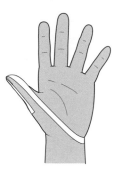

Figure 12.13

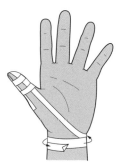

Figure 12.14

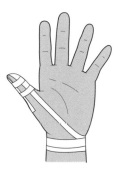

Figure 12.15

Tips

Inform the patient that adjustments may be made during the activity by pulling up the end of the tape and reapplying new tension around the wrist.

Simple thumb check-rein figure-of-eight method

R. Macdonald

INDICATION

Thumb hyperextension.

FUNCTION

To stabilize the joint and restrict extension and abduction of the thumb.

MATERIALS

2.5-cm or 1.25-cm tape.

POSITION

The hand is held in a functional position. (Face the operator to shake hands.)

APPLICATION

1. Start on the dorsal aspect of the proximal aspect of the thumb. Draw tape around the thumb towards the palm, then through the web, twisting the tape. Continue over the dorsal aspect of the hand, moulding the tape to the skin, then around and across the palmar surface to web moulding tape to the palm.
2. Draw the thumb towards the palm into a functional position and attach the tape to the starting point (do not wind the end around the thumb) (Fig. 12.16).

Apply this check rein over any thumb tape job.

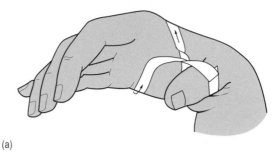

(a)

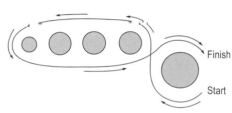

Finish

Start

(b)

Figure 12.16

Notes

To control extension – apply tension towards the palmar surface.
To control abduction – apply tension towards the dorsal surface.

Tips

Use adhesive spray on the palm of the hand for better adhesion, and
mould adhesive mass to the palm.
Check circulation by pressing the thumb nail.

Thumb spica taping

K.E. Wright

INDICATION

Thumb sprain.

FUNCTION

To provide support and stability for the first metacarpophalangeal joint of the hand.

MATERIAL

2.5-cm adhesive tape.

POSITION

Hand in palm-down position, with the thumb slightly flexed and the phalanges adducted.

APPLICATION

1. Apply an anchor strip of adhesive tape around the wrist (Fig. 12.17). Start at the ulnar condyle, cross the dorsal aspect of the distal forearm and encircle the wrist.
2. Apply the first of three support strips for the first metacarpophalangeal joint (Fig. 12.18). Starting at the ulnar condyle, cross the dorsum of the hand, cover the lateral joint line, encircle the thumb, proceed across the palmar aspect of the hand and finish at the ulnar condyle (Fig. 12.19).
3. Repeat step 2 twice (Fig. 12.20).
4. To help hold this procedure in place, apply a final anchor strip around the wrist (Fig. 12.21).

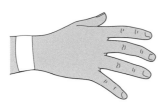

Figure 12.17

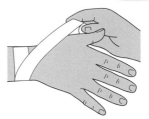

Figure 12.18

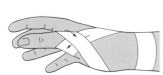

Figure 12.19

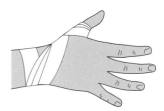

Figure 12.20

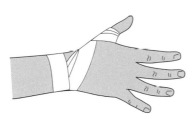

Figure 12.21

13

chapter

Spicas and triangular bandages

R. Macdonald

The spica or figure-of-eight bandage is very useful for a variety of conditions and can often be self-applied. In some situations, the spica is more appropriate than tape and is often used as a first-aid measure to protect the injured structure, to restrict range of motion and to minimize swelling and bleeding (Figs 13.1–13.6). Elastic stretch tape or any type of non-adhesive bandage may be used. If the support is to be removed for the application of cold or heat or therapeutic exercise, then a bandage is more appropriate as it may be used many times and is less costly. The spica must be applied firmly but not too tightly, each strip overlapping the previous one by half. A cold, wet spica is ideal for an acute injury. After application, check circulation and neural transmission.

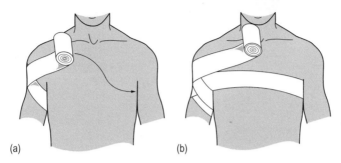

Figure 13.1 (a) and (b) Shoulder spica.

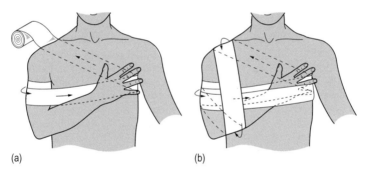

Figure 13.2 (a) and (b) Bandage to support a dislocation of the acromioclavicular and/or shoulder joint.

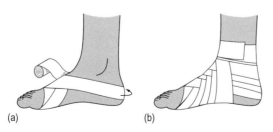

Figure 13.3 (a) and (b) Ankle and foot spica.

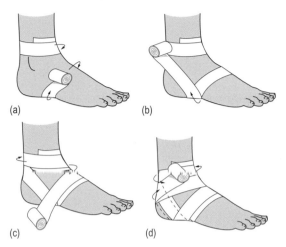

Figure 13.4 (a–d) Ankle wrap.

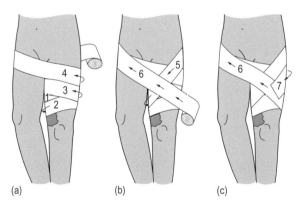

Figure 13.5 (a–c) Elastic groin support.

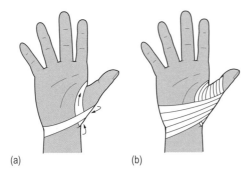

(a)   (b)

Figure 13.6 (a) and (b) Thumb spicas.

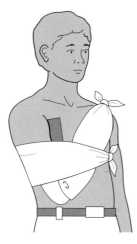

Figure 13.7 A sling for a fractured collarbone. Reproduced by kind permission of St John Ambulance. © Copyright 2003.

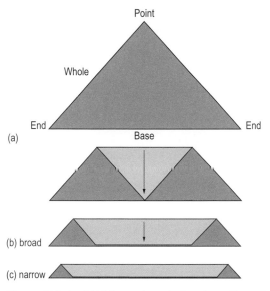

(a)
Point

Whole

End   End
Base

(b) broad

(c) narrow

Figure 13.8 (a–c) Folding a triangular bandage. Reproduced by kind permission of St John Ambulance. © Copyright 2003.

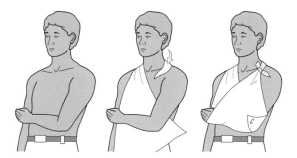

Figure 13.9 (a–c) Preparing an arm sling. Reproduced by kind permission of St John Ambulance. © Copyright 2003.

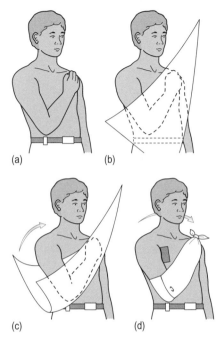

(a)

(b)

(c)

(d)

Figure 13.10 (a–d) Preparing an elevation sling. Reproduced by kind permission of St John Ambulance. © Copyright 2003.

Abduction	movement away from the midline of the body
Achilles tendon	tendon behind the heel
AC joint	acromioclavicular joint
Adduction	movement towards the midline of the body
Adhesive mass	sticky backing on tape
ADL	activities of daily living
Anterior	front
Anterior cruciate ligament	within the knee joint, limits anterior movement of the tibia on the femur
Assess	evaluate
Biceps	muscle on the front of the upper arm
Calcaneum	heel bone
Check rein	reinforced tape to restrict movement
Cohesive bandage	rubberized, sticks to itself and not to the skin
Condyle	bony end of the thigh bone
Contract	tense
Contralateral	opposite side
Contusion	bruise
Digit	finger/toe
Distal	area away from the centre of body or the furthest attachment
Dorsal	back (e.g. of the hand)
Extension	to straighten
Extensor tendons	on the front of the ankle joint

Femur	thigh bone
Flexion	to bend
Friction	rubbing
Hamstring	muscle at the back of the thigh
Hyperextend	to extend beyond the normal
Hypoallergenic	will not cause reaction on sensitive skin
Inferior	below
Innominate bones	flat bones that form the pelvic girdle
Inversion	turning in (e.g. ankle sprain)
Ipsilateral	same side
Kinesiology	study of motion of the human body
Lateral	side away from the body, outside
Ligaments	taut bands of tissue which bind bones together
Longitudinal arch	from heel to toes on the undersurface of the foot
Malleolus	ankle bone
Medial	side closest to the body, inside
MTSS	medial tibial stress syndrome
Palmar	front (e.g. of the hand)
Patella	knee cap
Pes cavus	foot with high rigid arch
Pes planus	foot with flat longitudinal arch
Peritendonitis	inflammation of the tendon sheath
Plantar fascia	tough bands of tissue on the sole of the foot
Plantar fasciitis	inflammation at the origin of the plantar fascia (near heel)
Plantarflex	toes and foot pointed downwards, towards the floor
Popliteal fossa	space behind the knee
Posterior	behind, rear
Pronate	turn palm down
Pronated feet	flat feet

Prone	lying face down
Proprioception	awareness of body position, perception of movement and change of direction
Proximal	close to the centre of the body or the nearest attachment
Quadriceps	muscles at the front of the thigh
Rehabilitate	to treat and restore to normal health
Rotator cuff	stabilizing muscles for the shoulder
Spica	figure-of-eight bandage technique
Sprain	overstretching or tearing of a ligament
SSTM	specific soft tissue massage
Strain	overstretching or tearing of a muscle
Superior	above
Supinate	turn palm up
Supine	lying on the back, facing upward
Tendinosis	degeneration in the tendon itself
Thenar eminence	muscular area of the thumb on the palm of the hand (intrinsic muscles)
Tibia	shin bone
Tibial tubercle	tibial attachment for the patellar tendon
Transverse arch	from medial to lateral
Valgus	distal bone/part pointing away from the midline of the body, knock knees
Varus	distal bone/part pointing toward the midline of the body, bow legs

Index

B

C

D

E

F

W

Waterproof tape, 5
Watson's strap, 134–5
Wrist, 178–91
  hyperextension injury, 188–9
  hyperflexion injury, 188–9
  inferior radioulnar joint taping,
    190–1